COVID

THE POLITICS
OF FEAR
AND THE POWER
OF SCIENCE

Turner Publishing Company
Nashville, Tennessee
www.turnerpublishing.com

Covid: The Politics of Fear and the Power of Science

Cover design: Rebecca Lown

Library of Congress Cataloging-in-Publication Data Upon Request

9781684426867 Hardcover
9781684426874 eBook

Printed in the United States of America

20 21 22 23 24   10 9 8 7 6 5 4 3 2 1

COVID

THE POLITICS OF FEAR AND THE POWER OF SCIENCE

Marc Siegel, M.D.

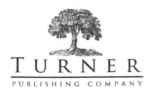

TURNER
PUBLISHING COMPANY

CONTENTS

PREFACE

On the 27th of January, 2020, I warned my TV viewers about a virus that had originated in Wuhan and spread to several other countries, with five reported cases in the United States at the time. "I've been studying contagions for a really long time, and I've never seen anything like this," I said. At the time, the Chinese government was reporting that at least 106 deaths had been attributed to the coronavirus, with more than 4,500 confirmed cases in the country. The state department urged Americans to reconsider traveling to Wuhan and ordered all non-emergency U.S. personnel and their families to leave China immediately. I called China's delay in imposing quarantines and travel restrictions "reckless and really, really scary," and indicated that I felt that the actual number of cases in China was far greater than was being reported. I also brought into question the role of the World Health Organization in obscuring the truth about the emerging pandemic and irresponsibly calling it a regional problem only.

Unfortunately, the information coming out of China proved to be unreliable and, in many cases, inaccurate. Meanwhile China restricted internal travel but continued to allow international travel including to Europe (where the virus soon spread).

Not only did we learn too late that you could easily acquire this virus from asymptomatic carriers and patients right before they developed symptoms (the rationale for increased mask use and enforced social distancing), but we also had to learn, here in New York City on very ill patients that this was a multi-organ inflammatory disease that often caused blood clotting and a vasculitis.

It also became clear how important travel bans in advance of the virus taking root were, since once this transmissible virus was in your community it would continue to spread despite lockdowns. New Zealand understood this better than perhaps any other country, and instituted an almost total travel ban that has kept the case numbers close to zero for months.

Here in the U.S. and elsewhere, lockdown had a tremendous economic, physical, and emotional cost, as routine medical care was delayed, jobs lost, and depression and suicidal thoughts soared, especially among our young, who were out of work or out of school, living in a state of relative isolation.

Any attempt to put this pandemic in proper medical context was immediately overcome by politics. The virus itself humbled us the more we learned about it. Here in the U.S., it ravaged New York first, hitting the media nerve directly, and our suffering was felt everywhere as this respiratory virus ravaged us before moving on. Would the cold weather bring it back? We learned that it was a wildly contagious virus that caused inflammatory sequelae. It inflamed the inside of blood vessels and could damage the lungs, the heart, the brain, and other organs. It was hard to dismiss most cases as being mild when it turned out that some people went undiagnosed until a mental fog or fatigue or shortness of breath persisted (known as long haulers). This virus preyed on the defenseless, ravaging defenseless nursing homes most of all. Daily case numbers were trumpeted by the *New York Times* and the *Washington Post*, the slowly decreasing number of hospitalizations or deaths were obscured.

Mask wars ruled; those who believed they offered almost complete protection from this virus and those who insisted on the personal freedom not to wear them, despite the risk. And the freedom to protest racial injustice was positioned versus the freedom to attend a presidential rally or attend a church gathering, all events risking spread of a virus if it were there in the crowd. Rioters looted and burned cars and buildings, definitely not socially distanced.

Of course, both passionate protesters or shouting ralliers were more likely to take few precautions, potentially spreading virus. Public health was supposed to triumph in all cases but gave way to political expediency. Meanwhile, the inexpensive arthritis drug hydroxychloroquine was attacked by the president's opponents because he praised it and then took it himself, before it was fully studied. Others swore by it despite the lack of proof. When news that an anti-viral drug, remdesivir, which cost thousands, had a moderate effect against COVID, the results were trumpeted beyond the actual real world use. The politics of fear obscured the science of a widely spreading virus which gummed up the health care system and interfered with life-saving treatments for cancer, heart disease, etc. As

Spring gave way to Summer and Summer to Fall, heedless young people spread the virus, putting older or sicker people at risk. There was the hope of a new, cheap rapid accurate antigen test for screening that was due to be distributed widely, and there was growing hope for a vaccine, meanwhile, there were large outbreaks at college campuses. The presidential election polarized everything to the nth degree. The Republican National Convention took place on the lawn of the White House with nary a mask or physically distant attendee or COVID test in sight. And the unruly riots that broke out afterward seemed more likely to spread the virus if there was any in the crowds. And though the Democratic National Convention took place virtually, at the same time, the Democrats supported the cheek-to-jowl protests. The rule of the day was the politics of fear and intimidation trumping the absolute need for public health. As we approached the Fall, we remained in a dark place in America, with many of our restaurants, theaters, schools and workplaces still shuttered, awaiting the promise of a vaccine, and with only physical distancing and masking and personal hygiene to protect us. There were many COVID treatments in the pipeline, but there was nothing for prevention or early treatment that we can all agree on. We needed to stop all the finger pointing and ridiculing, and replace all the dogma and self-righteousness with kindness and respect, with courage instead of fear, but that wasn't so easy for such a politically divided nation.

If you read this story in a novel you would not believe it was really happening, and you would find it impossible to predict the ending.

INTRODUCTION

This book was originally conceived almost twenty years ago, unexpectedly, during a southbound trip on the FDR Drive in New York City on the morning of September 11, 2001. It was a bright, hot morning when I began to notice the multicolored ambulances from all over the city—Columbia Presbyterian, Metropolitan, St. Vincent's—traveling alongside and passing me, all exiting at Bellevue Hospital.

I volunteered my services to the transforming emergency center at Bellevue that morning, absorbing the rush of human emotion—at once committed to the task and yet frightened. The fact that ultimately there weren't the survivors to fill our beds did little to stem the fright. People worked to keep their minds off the unfolding disaster, and this, I discovered, was a necessary coping strategy.

As I volunteered my services to the Red Cross and to my patients in the succeeding months, I discovered a newfound vulnerability. I entered the media world and found that each health care topic I discussed in an article or on TV seemed blown out of proportion to the real danger. I seized the chance to learn about each succeeding "bug du jour" and to try to offer perspective and a salve of reassurance whenever I could.

We all personalized 9/11, and it made us all feel more at risk, whether we were really at risk or not. We grew afraid more easily than before, misinformed by our leaders and provoked by the news media.

We have never been the same since.

Anthrax was the first manifestation in concrete terms of this personalized susceptibility. I was honored to participate in a U.S. Senate investigation into the handling of the anthrax crisis, directed by Senator Chuck Grassley of Iowa. I discovered amidst the CDC and U.S. Postal Service papers and letters to and from the senator a sense of fumbling. Fear out of proportion to the real risks was made worse by a lack of preparedness. Even if you didn't have a reason to be afraid before, you could see how poorly you would be protected if there really were a reason to fear.

During the health care scares of the next few years, my patients shared their fears with me every day. I would never have been able to conceive of fear in real terms if it weren't for their willingness to share their concerns and experiences.

I witnessed their fear of SARS, despite the fact that I never saw any evidence that SARS was close to becoming widespread. My office phone rang with anxieties over influenza as it went from being a ho-hum underappreciated killer to the latest rage.

I understood from the outset that our fear mechanism had gone awry, but I didn't know exactly how. I could study the process by which dangers were manufactured and provoked, but as a medical doctor I also had to study the original fight-or-flight mechanism that was intended to protect us. The place to start was with animals.

FEAR INVADED OUR homes like never before, affecting more and more people. Newspaper headlines were apocalyptic warnings. Media obsessions fueled our cycles of worry, which burned out only to be replaced by more alarming cycles.

The passions and routines of everyday life were our primary defenses against this contagious fear. These defenses, however, were being eroded, bombarded by the ongoing doom-and-gloom of the daily news, until they were completely hijacked by COVID-19, and there was no everyday life anymore. But twenty-four hours of cable news continued to infiltrate our sleep, and was almost as damaging to our health as cigarette smoke was to our defenses against cancer.

How did it get to be this way? Fear was looming larger in our lives now with the pandemic more than ever before. Yet no one had ever tried to integrate what scientists had learned about the physiology of fear with the increased reliance on fear on the part of both the media and the politicians. Of course, some fears had their origin in real events, most prominently the attacks of September 11, 2001, and now, the spread of the coronavirus, which at the time of this writing had already infected more than 6 million people in the U.S. alone, killing close to 200,000. Still, despite the real ever-present danger from COVID, the overall climate of fear was inflated well out of proportion to the risk and the reality and was its own core danger to society.

My investigations of fear showed me that it is designed to be protective, that animals use it to sense genuine threats to their survival. At the same time, humans have the ability to exaggerate fear until it threatens our health.

Under the stress of unremitting fear, we have become more susceptible to disease, including heart disease, stroke, and cancer. Once we become sick, our fear grows. In my medical practice I dealt with many patients who were so alarmed by their illness that even offering an effective treatment wasn't enough to reassure them. In treating this fear, and in analyzing health scares in my columns and on television, I tried to uncover the moment of lost perspective when dangers were first distorted.

My investigation of fear began with the discovery that animals respond by instinct and conditioning, while we, with the same essential fear apparatus as them, feed our fears through verbal communication. A zebra is wise to be afraid of a roaring lion, yet we are not so wise to fear a metaphorical lion that is a thousand miles away from us. As soon as we hear about a danger, however remote, we tend to see it as a personal threat, especially if the danger is exaggerated from the beginning.

This pattern of distortion led me directly to the media. How many of us listen to somber-toned newscasters and expect that what we are hearing is valid information? Many of us grew up believing we could find truth in the news. When did the crew-cut, thick-glasses, thin-tie anchorman become today's harbinger of doom?

Media people I meet are often serious and sincere, which doesn't mean they always see risk in a proper context. Newspapers issue daily corrections, but do not routinely acknowledge when threats are reported that don't materialize or when real threats like COVID become gradually better.

In studying fear, I came to believe that it has a tendency to reignite itself. Once a fear fire is extinguished another one takes its place. There are fear seekers in our society, and there are plenty of worriers in between.

When it comes to the fear epidemic, are Americans unique? In parts of the world where wars and acts of terrorism are more commonplace, America has the reputation of being a country with a soft underbelly.

In Israel most people manage to live relatively normal lives despite frequent suicide bombings and constant military conflict. COVID became just another dangerous occurrence. People there understand that statistically, a walk to the supermarket is still far more likely to be uneventful than unsafe, and the public has come to understand and accept the small level of individual risk.

Still, even in Israel the daily threats have a cumulative effect on health. Suicide bombings that occur one year have an impact on the perceived sense of safety the next year.

It is not necessary to have a psychiatric disorder in order to be made ill by fear. This is the essential distinction between the well-described diagnoses of anxiety and phobia and the new fear disease that can victimize anyone. And superimposing fears on a population that is already riddled with phobias and anxieties can induce paralysis.

Imagine how someone who was afraid of flying felt after being saturated by the media images of September 11. Or someone who was already afraid of COVID because a neighbor had it, felt when bombarded by images of COVID non-stop on TV.

The symptoms of fear, the maladaptive kind, include an exaggerated sense of vulnerability, out of proportion to the actual risk. Like any illness, the illness of fear interferes with function. Fear victims are revved up in fight-or-flight mode. Their bodies ask them, how is a person to be protected from an ever-growing threat without being on the alert? Stress hormones—adrenaline, catecholamines, and cortisol—are secreted in excess amounts. These counter-regulatory hormones cause the liver to make more sugar and create more and more energy, which builds up without proper outlet. To this, nervous sedentary people add more stimulants such as coffee, which revs them up further. It is a perfect storm. People don't eat well, sleep well, or experience sufficient pleasure because they are always on the alert.

Why such an easy path to hysteria? For months I pored through books and articles trying to figure this out. The tiny pecan-shaped organ deep in the center of all animal brains—the amygdala—serves as the central station for processing fear. Once it has been triggered, the amygdala is difficult to stop. Fear learning and fear memories are stored in the pre-frontal cortex which is hard wired to the amygdala. The higher centers that help you to unlearn fear are weak by comparison and easily overrun by fear memory.

Beyond our animal instincts, for many of us our Judeo-Christian background makes fear a familiar concept that can easily motivate us. A disapproving God, we learn, is ready to punish us. Postmodern panic may have its origins in the collective memory of biblical scourges.

With fear infecting and reinfecting us, our pill-happy culture looks for quick treatments for our fears. Whether this pill is propranolol, Valium, Prozac, or another brew, we believe that without it, we will be compelled to live in terror. Rather than examine why we are unnecessarily afraid, rather than rip out this weed of fear by its roots, we attempt to neutralize it with postmodern concoctions.

In addition to pills, we seek the ultimate fear vaccine. In a study from Israel in May 2004, Jonathan Kipnis gave a chemical cocktail to panicked mice and found that by bolstering their beleaguered neurons, the mice were once again able to perform their usual tasks. The implication of these results—if they prove applicable to humans—is that immunologically engineered "vaccines" may one day help to make people impervious to panic. But it is one thing to employ sophisticated technologies to bolster an overworked nerve fiber in a troubled brain, it is another to bottle the latest preventative and market it widely to treat all fear. Instead of learning how to assess risk realistically, we are quick to try to treat fear with the latest in immunology.

Traditional vaccines already provide us with an apparent shield against our fear of illness. During the summer of 2020, many of us reassured ourselves with the thought of a coming coronavirus vaccine long before large scale testing had begun. But it may well be another media creation to believe that a simple inoculation removes all risk.

The public pendulum swings from dependency on a supposed panacea to panic when a vaccine is found to be flawed or is not readily available. The government makes fear a central part of its agenda, trying to weigh in as our protector. In the process of being so "protected," we learn about dangers we didn't know existed. The real danger of being manipulated in this way is to our health.

I first learned of the devastating reach of governmental fear mongering when, at the request of Senator Chuck Grassley, I examined the response to the 2001 anthrax mailings. The Centers for Disease Control (CDC), back then, attached itself to the media megaphone and made us all feel afraid to open our mail. This response was a way of covering up the miscommunication and mishandling of the evidence by all the federal agencies involved.

The anthrax scare established a precedent for public health hysteria that was racheted up with each new *bug du jour*, to the point where the public felt threatened by every possible source of contagion. Smallpox extended the hype to a bug that was no longer infecting anyone. SARS was the first panic to involve the worldwide health community, and petrify Asia and Canada along with the United States. The bird flu scare turned an overlooked disease into a sensation overnight. Swine flu, the new pandemic in 2009, was a new pathogen and was worthy of our concern, but it ended up being a relatively mild virus which we were far too fearful to predict. Ebola, in 2014, was incredibly deadly, but media and political hype obscured its poor transmissibility, and then, tragically, as soon as it was over we forgot all about pandemic preparedness and, so, were unprepared for the massive COVID-19 pandemic. And even though this sickened many millions around the world, and would kill more than a million, our fears outpaced even the virus as our society shut down at tremendous cost.

The government is sometimes a greater danger than the supposed threat. In its haste to protect us from chemical and biological weapons, for example, the government built expensive high-security laboratories to study these potential weapons. But a study published in February 2001 found that of twenty-one known germ attacks, most were conducted not by terrorists, but by government researchers-turned-terrorists who had gained access to human pathogens.

And then there is the "elephant in the room" our leaders practically have ignored the risk of nuclear terrorism, where a terrorist smuggling a suitcase onto a plane or boat could get past the porous safety net and cause great harm. As Harvard scholar Graham Allison wrote in his book, *Nuclear Terrorism*, "this was one worst-case scenario we weren't doing nearly enough to try to prevent."

Perhaps our greatest immunity against panic has always come from go-to people in charge of our safety: the policemen, firefighters, and emergency medical technicians. But these comforting presences have been forced to compete with the all-purpose information glut. Tiny bites of data are always within reach via the Internet, the television, social media and the radio. Many of my patients complain that they don't know where to go to find answers that don't frighten them. Our personal narratives are giving way more and more to the discourse of risk and danger.

We believe that strangers are a threat to us, but as Barry Glassner, the author of *The Culture of Fear*, pointed out, most crimes involve people known to the victim.

Some of the narratives of this book are drawn from the many patients I have known who have lived in fear and have struggled to cope in the face of growing misinformation. Their stories are juxtaposed with the true science that has eluded them and the societal trends that have heightened their anxiety.

Despite the growing fear, there are those who have developed hard reflexes to cope with real dangers. Emergency workers are trained to put their own risks in perspective. Firefighters can not function if they are afraid of being burned or overcome by smoke, and doctors have to put aside their fear of catching a patient's illness in order to do their jobs. I learned this on the job as an intern and resident battling HIV in my patients, but this has never been more true than with COVID. This training required a concentrated effort.

A social plan for stabilizing public hysteria involves countering false beliefs regarding danger. But fear researchers have determined that seeing fear in practical terms is far from easy.

In examining and reexamining fear, I have attempted to find a new social model to explain today's COVID pandemic. Using my tools as an internist, I have discovered that the disease model for infection and epidemic fits fear the best. Fear is physiological, but today's fear had become pathological. It spread via distorted hype to those who might not have been overly worried in the first place.

We build up a partial immunity to each cycle of fear with the simple passage of time. We become desensitized, and we learn that the threat we have been coached to fear is not likely to occur or reoccur. But fear is not easily unlearned. It buries itself in our brain's pre-frontal cortex. Our deep emotions can override our reason at any time.

Groundbreaking animal studies by Dr. Esther Sabban showed that once frightened, an animal is more susceptible to the next threat that comes along. Fear memory, like all the powerful emotions deep in our brains, is hard for us to overcome or outreason.

Fear has become pervasive. In order to eradicate it, we have to first understand it from the microscopic level all the way to the larger issues of national defense and public safety. In examining fear, I have attempted to use my understanding of health and disease as a lens to spot the epidemic as it is spreading and infecting more and more people. I begin with the biology, move on to the personal, and then widen my lens to the systemic.

To understand why our society's hysteria has grown, I have found it is important to look at the individual. I try to determine why a person's physiology can turn so quickly to pathology.

Our fear biology can wear us down rather than protect us. Fear deeply affects individual patients, from physical illness all the way to imagined terrorism. The government, media, and private businesses contribute to the perpetual pressure to be afraid.

Publicly reported infections contribute to a growing climate of panic.

There is an important border between religion and superstition, and there is a link between hypochondria, anxiety, and common fear. I have grown certain that unnecessary fear is harmful and can be eliminated.

In my life, in treating my patients, and in studying fear, I have found that one effective treatment for fear is to replace it with another deep emotion, like caring. If a person develops a passion that takes her or him beyond a self-absorbing cycle of worry, this passion can be used to breed the antithesis of fear, also known as courage.

Sixteen years ago, my three-year-old daughter, Rebecca, fractured her thigh bone in a fall. For several days after the cast was removed and an X-ray showed that the bone had healed, she remained afraid to walk on it. Finally, during an exciting time at the beach she stood on the sand and watched the waves come in. By the time fear memory got ready to extend its shadowy tentacles, it was too late—she was already placing weight on the healed leg. Once Rebecca experienced the reward of renewed mobility, she was able to neutralize her fear. Sixteen years later she went through the same process when she finally learned to ride a bicycle.

Even in the midst of COVID, those with courage or passion might be able to stand up to fear arising from real, yet over-personalized dangers. If enough people develop courage, this immunized group can slow the spread of fear through their community in the same way that those who have been vaccinated slow the spread of any contagion.

ONE NIGHT I received a text from a good friend named Ashley, I hadn't heard from her in several months. She had moved to another network, but we had stayed in touch.

"Can you get me a prescription," she wrote.

"For what?" my reply.

My friend didn't answer me directly, but texted back that she had type A positive blood type. She had never asked me for a prescription before. It took me a moment to puzzle this out.

"Were you exposed to COVID?"

"No."

"You want hydroxychloroquine? Why?"

"You are seeing patients. You should be taking it too."

I texted back that the treatment was unproven, and though I felt it still had potential as a preventive or for early treatment as I was discussing on TV, (she knew that my 96-year-old father had been given the prescription by his cardiologist when he'd developed a sudden cough, fever, and fatigue back in March), I didn't think either of us should be taking it. Studies were ongoing. This seemed to calm my friend slightly, though I was struck by the extent of her fear. She had a young child at home, and she, like everyone else, was massively afraid of the pandemic and was both fixating on her personal risk as she saw it through a fear lens, reaching for quick and easy solutions to provide calm.

"There are also no real studies showing that your blood type is really associated with more severe cases. That's just conjecture and myth at this point. A new study from Harvard showed no association." "Whew," she wrote back instantly. "So glad to hear that." The science of fear predicts that the worse a threat becomes the more we will over-personalize it and reach for non-scientific solutions. The more invisible and microscopic the danger, the more unpredictable and widespread, the more it will be underestimated initially and then whipped and flogged by a news media anxious for attention and ratings, and by inconsistent politicians thirsty for votes, and the worse our fears will become.

FEAR HAS A powerful effect on the human brain. A complex network of neural connections lodges fear memories in the pre-frontal cortex. Fear is a strong emotion that easily overrides our higher centers of reason. We think we are risk assessing, when instead we are constantly driven by irrational fears. We inherit this mechanism from our animal forbears. The amygdala in the center of the brain triggers an outpouring of stress hormones in response to a perceived danger. Fear memories are engaged which bring us back to our earliest perils.

Our emotional brain struggles for answers and so we engage in what I call A + B = D type thinking. So it was with COVID: (A) there was a wildly spreading virus out there that could kill any one of us and cause long term problems even from mild cases. (B) It could reside on surfaces and even hang in the air for several minutes especially indoors in places with poor ventilation. (D) We were all at risk all the time. Missing was (C), that even if asymptomatic spread or spread through casual contact was quite possible, we didn't know exactly how often that actually occurred, and meanwhile, the old tried and true method of respiratory viral spread—namely a sick person coughing or sneezing or even shouting in your vicinity was still what you needed to watch out for the most. Unfortunately, fear was never linear, and so as the pandemic progressed we dilated the improbable and it obfuscated the most likely.

This fear and uncertainty over spread and what to do about it led to a public war over masks. (A) The virus spread widely, and even mild cases, could lead to long term problems. (B) Masks offered protection against spread, though we didn't know how much. Masks appeared to be useful in other cultures where mask wearing was common. An observational study (not proof) at Massachusetts General Hospital showed that health care workers wearing masks routinely appeared to decrease the spread of COVID. Other studies were coming out including one at Nebraska Medicine which showed that cities that had mask mandates faired better than those that didn't. (D) Everyone had to wear masks in public at all times. Missing was (C), the scientific proof that masks always worked, whether they were worn properly, or even when they were worn loosely, or changed infrequently, or when they were used instead of social distancing.

One group believed that masks rendered them practically invulnerable against the virus. This group clung to masks as a form of religion while COVID-shaming the other group who lived in denial and rejected masks entirely. There was no debate or real discussion about masks, only the religious dogma and the heretics who rebelled against it. One shocking example of this occurred in Bayonne, France, on July 5th, 2020 when a French bus diver was beaten to death by passengers who refused to wear face masks. The more the virus spread, the more foolish the mask-haters looked and the more justified the mask-lovers appeared, especially as more and more population studies showed mask effectiveness at decreasing viral spread, and providing some protection not just for others from the mask wearers, but also likely for the mask wearer against incoming respiratory virus. Despite the actual science, in the end, both groups were driven by their emotions.

Masks were one prop against our fear. Another was treatment. (A) We were struggling to find an early treatment to protect ourselves. (B)

Hydroxychloroquine had been shown to have some anti-viral affect against this SARS COV 2 virus, and studies done in France and at the Henry Ford Hospital System in Detroit appeared to back this up while several other studies had shown the opposite. (D) Hydroxychloroquine should be discarded and its proponents (including President Trump) mocked.

Missing of course was the scientific proof (C) we needed: Double blinded randomized studies—the gold standard—for early or prophylactic use were still in progress, though no one on either side of the political battle over this drug had the patience to wait, including my friend Ashley.

The pandemic led to fear and the fear led to the false comfort found in dogma. The dogma resulted in divisiveness which then stoked more fear.

Ill prepared and inconsistent leadership fanned the flames of our COVID fears. Back in March we became aware that the CDC, state and local health departments had dropped the ball on testing and the virus was spreading uncontrolled throughout our communities, especially here in New York. There was a striking shortage of diagnostic testing initially, and the meager tests the CDC did provide us were faulty. The PCR test we were relying on were developed in the 1990's and were somewhat cumbersome. The more efficient, less accurate rapid antigen testing we could use on entire populations wouldn't become available until at least September, when we were already several months into the pandemic. The lack of knowing who had the dreaded virus and who didn't, who was a carrier and who wasn't—all undermined our crucial need to contact trace, and spread unnecessary fear.

Looming shortages of ventilators and ICU beds and personal protective equipment were used to justify the severe lockdown to a petrified populace. Even if this approach was helpful at decreasing viral spread, there was a tremendous economic, emotional, and physical cost. The case and hospitalization numbers and the death rate all dropped dramatically by mid May. Fear-driven compliance clearly helped. The COVID surge in Texas, Florida, Arizona, and California that followed in July was different, as heedless maskless young people grouped together and spread the virus. Denial was another primary manifestation of fear, and could be quite destructive. Young people who had been locked down for too long rebelled by grouping together and spreading the virus. Reclosing bars and restaurants, gyms and hair salons, even cancelling elective surgeries were all justified. These moves slowed the onslaught of COVID-19 cases into hospitals and ICUs, but the economic and emotional cost was once again severe, not to mention the physical cost of delaying tests and treatments.

Public health measures required a sincere, unified message to maximize compliance. COVID-19 was a disaster of almost unprecedented proportions, which was all the more reason we needed fear leaders from the get-go to unify in order to properly inform and reassure us. Instead, political expediency divided us. The mask group (including Mayor DiBlasio of New York) excused protests (against the horrific murder of George Floyd and other police shootings) as a source of disease spread despite the lack of social distancing and even consistent mask use. This group used the fact that the virus was somewhat less likely to spread out of doors as a justification, while at the same time ridiculing President Trump's political rallies (which occurred indoors) as a high risk of spread. Even if this were true, it certainly didn't justify protests from a public health point of view. At the July protest in Detroit following the police shooting of Hakim Littleton, for example, there was no social distancing and barely a mask in sight.

Fear and division undermined the crucial question of whether or not to reopen our schools, even in areas where there was very little virus, despite the fact that: (1) Studies had shown that young children were probably less likely to get sick from COVID or to spread it to adults, though young people were still at some risk of longer term complications. (2) Countries throughout Europe had succeeded at various degrees of school re-openings without a corresponding increase in cases. Studies from Germany, France, Sweden, Switzerland and elsewhere confirmed this. (3) There was no evidence that children in school were more likely to spread COVID to higher risk groups, including the elderly, than when they were out of school. (4) The public health cost of keeping kids out of school was high. As Dr. Anthony Fauci, director of the National Institute of Allergy and Infectious Diseases said to me in an interview, "If you keep children out of school the unintended consequences can be profound, with regard to what do the parents do. Stay off from work to be able to take care of their children? What about child care? What about children who rely on their schools for their lunch? Maybe the most important nutritional meal that they'll get."

Indeed, schools had been reopening all over the world with positive results, and little or no virus spread. France gradually opened schools to younger children and then high schoolers, and in Denmark, Norway, Belgium, and all across Europe decisions were made successfully to reopen

schools with smaller classroom size. Only in Israel was there an outbreak tied to school reopening in a hot zone for COVID, and that had to do with relaxing guidelines.

Yet fear of the virus clouded decisions here on whether to reopen the schools, even when they were in areas of little or no virus, and this thinking extended to universities, despite the fact that they had built-in quarantine situations, in case anyone got sick. In fact, an entire university could be quarantined, and still continue to function. It was disappointing that Harvard, for example, despite the fact that there were very few cases of COVID in Massachusetts, elected to continue with online learning only, with less than half of its students residing on campus. This model quickly spread to many other universities around the country.

I approached Brown University, my alma mater, with a careful list of ideas on how best to reopen. Here is what I suggested: (1) testing and two weeks self-quarantine before arrival. (2) Brown chartered buses (or planes) sent out to pick up the students. (3) Retesting on arrival. (4) Temperature and symptom checks on entrance to all buildings. (5) Nurses and nurse practitioners stationed throughout the campus. (6) Weekly testing of all teachers and custodial personnel. (7) Isolation of anyone who is sick with suspected COVID.

Brown University President Christina Paxson praised my suggestions before ultimately rejecting them. I suspected that fear and internal politics predominated. Rhode Island was a state with very few cases and Brown was sequestered on the east side of Providence, which could be easily isolated if necessary. No one asked the professors or staff whether they would agree to hold regular classes, instead, Brown planned a hybrid schedule of online and in person, with no large lectures and a twelve month schedule so that classes and students could be spaced out. The core experience was gone, especially when they cancelled the hybrid in mid August and went to online only.

Thinking back, it was clear that our fears were attached to how rapidly and unexpectedly the virus had come at us in the first place. Amid reassurances from China and the World Health Organization, in early 2020 the Chinese government restricted travel to and from Wuhan, the epicenter, while at the same time not restricting travel to Europe, where the virus quickly spread. Our scientists were reassured when the structure of the virus was published online, but were not informed at how wildly

contagious it was or that it caused a blood clotting problem and inflammation not just in the lungs, but on the inside of blood vessels potentially affecting all the major organs in the body.

The origin of the virus was also shrouded in mystery, which petrified us. Political cries of xenophobia turned to true suspicion that we had been misinformed or lied to, a rare moment of bi-partisanship, though the political right was far more suspicious of the extent of the lie. Did the virus really originate in Wuhan, or did it accidentally infect someone at the nearby virology lab where "gain of function" experiments, supported by our own NIH, testing the capacity of a virus to infect humans, were being conducted.

During a trip to Dulles airport for Fox News in late February, I learned from Deputy Director of Homeland Security Ken Cuccinelli and a disturbed Custom and Border Protection agent just how easy it was for travelers to lie about symptoms or point of origin and slip back into the U.S. with COVID. I asked a woman wearing a mask at an Air China counter how she intended to get back into the U.S., and she said, "none of your business."

At the National Quarantine Center at Nebraska Medical Center I learned just how easily transmissible the virus was and I began to warn the public. But it was already too late. The viral horses were long out of the barn and we were overwhelmed by both virus and fear of virus.

By August 21st, 2020, Institute for Health Metrics and Evaluation (IHME) at the University of Washington predicted that the U.S. would reach 310,000 deaths by December 1, 2020, and that if mask wearing increased to 95%, more than 69,000 lives could be saved. The problem with mathematical projections like these, even from highly regarded groups like IHME, was that they were still based on speculation and automatically spread fear.

Fear terminology predominated throughout the Spring and Summer. The term "second wave" petrified us, as we anticipated an onslaught in the Fall, as the media failed to mention that origin of the term "second wave," was the 1918 Spanish flu, when it is believed that the virus mutated and became both more deadly and more contagious. So far it appeared that this coronavirus had done neither.

We also became more afraid of the impact of the virus itself as it became clearer and clearer that it caused damage to many other organs in the body besides just the lungs. Blood clots were common, and one cohort German study showed a high percentage of patients (78%) with heart inflammation (myocarditis) after the acute illness, which was frequently mild. Autopsy studies confirmed heart involvement in many patients.

And then a scary term began to surface known as "long haulers." A significant percentage of patients, many who had mild symptoms to begin with, ended up with longer term complications including lung or heart damage. So it was now wrong to suggest that it was okay if young people spread COVID as long as high risk or older people didn't get it, since some ended up with long term perhaps even permanent problems.

The one unified hope against our fears was the potential vaccine. People everywhere grasped the exciting concepts that several candidates were in play, that most utilized brand new genetic technologies (messenger RNA) or viral protein delivery systems (an adenovirus particle from a chimpanzee or human), and that over the summer three of these vaccines were already entering late stage clinical trials and had a shot of being ready for use by the end of the year. People on both sides of the political aisle shared the excitement over the manufacturing scheme where all liability and cost were absorbed by the government and production was being geared up to match the science. This approach had never been used before in history, and if it succeeded millions of lives would be saved.

All of us could agree on the importance of a working vaccine. Many began to see it as a fulcrum for the fight against both the virus and the fear it generated. If we managed to get a vaccine, it could bring us all together, even as it immunized us against both the coronavirus and our fear of the virus. Were we putting all our hopes prematurely in one untested basket? Yes we were.

Should we be more afraid of the virus or the vaccine we produced to protect us against it? That had always been the question. Overall, vaccines were the greatest public health accomplishments of the 20th and the 21st century, though in 1976 a military recruit at Fort Dix dying from an emerging strain of swine flu brought up the specter of the 1918 pandemic and there was a rush to a vaccine. Unfortunately, this vaccine was linked to close to a thousand cases of Guillan Barre Syndrome and was hastily withdrawn.

But not before someone very close to me had received the vaccine, something that I was only made aware of very recently.

"I haven't been the same since," my 96 year old father said, "and there is no way I will be first in line for this vaccine either. You and the president can go before me," he said, referring to my interview with President Trump where we agreed to both take the new vaccine when it became available—at the same time.

"What happened in 1976?"

"I was in bed after that for several days."

"Did you have ascending paralysis?"

"No. I was in a fog. I couldn't think straight. I couldn't put my thoughts together and my memory went. I haven't been the same since."

"Encephalopathy. Brain swelling. Are you sure it was the vaccine?"

"No question. Ever since, I have waited a year or more before I will try a new vaccine."

I had to admit that I had the same policy, not because I had ever sustained side effects, but because while several thousand were tested with a new vaccine, it wasn't until the first year of use that millions were given it and the results on a mass scale could really be assessed.

With the pandemic, I was more afraid of the virus than of a new vaccine, but I had to admit the technology was very new and untested. There was still a lot that could go wrong.

A vaccine had never been produced at this rate of speed before. The measles vaccine had taken several years.

Operation Warp Speed, a revolutionary program developed by the Trump administration, was matching manufacturing with the science, so that there wouldn't be a delay between the emergence of an effective vaccine and its approval by the FDA, scaled up production, and distribution. In fact, by August, billions of dollars had already been given out to support several vaccine candidates as they entered later stage trials, where each vaccine was tested in around 30,000 people. Pfizer/BioNTech, Moderna, Oxford University/Astra Zeneca, Novavax, and Johnson & Johnson each received over a billion dollars for vaccine production. The technology in each case was different, with Moderna and the BioNTech vaccine utilizing what was known as a messenger RNA platform: A strand of encoded genetic material messages to our cells to produce the same spike protein that the SARS COV2 virus has on its surface and allows it to invade our cells. Our immune system responds to this protein by making neutralizing antibodies and powerful immune hunters known as T cells.

Both Messenger RNA vaccines showed strong immune responses and both were generally well tolerated with the exception of temporary symptoms of headache, fever, muscle aches, or fatigue. They also showed immunity against challenges of the virus in non-human primates. But it remained to be seen how effective they would be at preventing infection in humans.

This was the primary purpose of Phase 3 trials, which were launched over the summer.

The Oxford vaccine, by contrast, relied on a chimpanzee adenovirus vector (stripped of its ability to make you ill) carrying a genetic payload which also provoked the cells to produce the spike protein found on SARS COV 2. It too had been shown effective and safe in early clinical trials.

The novavax vaccine also involved an introduction of the spike protein (grown in giant vats of insect cells) and in early trials appeared to have an immune response (neutralizing antibody) four times that of people recovering from COVID-19.

Russia, meanwhile, approved another adenovirus vector vaccine from the renowned Gamaleya Institute for use in high risk groups against the coronavirus, after it had been tried in only 76 people, a reckless move that deeply disturbed scientists around the world. Fear of the virus and fear of the government were combined. Still, the plan was not to use it widely until January, after large scale clinical trials were completed.

And China too was far along with their own vaccine candidates, especially the CanSino adenovirus vaccine, which was also in late stage clinical trials over the summer and had potential to be released by the end of the year.

The closer the science got to a vaccine that could slow the spread of the SARS COV 2 virus around the world, the more people spoke about it and relied on the concept. If successful, it would be an unprecedented accomplishment in human history.

Coronavirus vaccines existed for animals, and early vaccine trials had taken place for SARS and MERS, two earlier coronaviruses that had limited outbreaks. Fear of the virus was so widespread around the world, it was unlikely that it would be fully replaced by fear of a new high tech vaccine, though there was certain to be non-compliance among anti-vaxxers, and those, like my father, who had personal memories of the 1976 swine flu vaccine fiasco. But it was fear which divided us far more than any virus could. We needed to come together in order to defeat it, and in the process, with the help of a new vaccine, we might vanquish the virus too.

PART ONE

PRE-COVID

FIGHT OR FLIGHT

"We cannot wait while dangers gather."

—Condoleezza Rice, then national security adviser,
addressing the 9/11 Commission on April 8, 2004

WHY ARE WE SO AFRAID?

Fear has been with humankind from the beginning and is part of our psychological makeup from birth. Our earliest fears are tied to Mommy disappearing even for an instant, taking away our only comfort and protection. Children are afraid of the unknown. It is only as they develop that they learn to distinguish a sense of global uncertainty from a specific danger.

As we become adults, our fears are tied to specific threats, an association that distinguishes fear from anxiety. Anxiety can be self-perpetuating, as it often originates in neurosis or self-doubt. Anxious people worry when they don't need to. Fear, on the other hand, is meant to be an essential tool. We have inherited the fear apparatus, practically unchanged, from our animal forebears, but we often allow it to generate self-defeating hysteria.

When fear is unremitting, especially when it is constantly provoked but no protective action can be taken, anxiety and hysteria often result.

"You're absolutely fine," I said to my patient who couldn't catch her breath.

"No, I'm not," she insisted, coughing and wheezing.

It was only when she told me that her wedding was the following weekend that I saw her fear turning to anxiety, and decided to forgo an extensive lung workup.

THE BIOLOGY OF FEAR

Fear is more than a state of mind; it's chemical. It is present in the circuitry of our brains, in the neurochemical exchanges between nerves. Fear is a physical reaction to a perceived threat. As long as the danger is direct and real, fear is normal and helps to protect us.

When an individual feels threatened, fear revs up the metabolism in anticipation of an imminent need to defend oneself or flee. "Fight or flight," or the "acute stress response," was first described by Walter Cannon, an American physiologist, in the 1920s. Cannon observed that animals, including humans, react to threats with a hormonal discharge of the nervous system. There is an outpouring of vessel-constricting, heart-thumping hormones, including noradrenaline (norepinephrine) and adrenaline (epinephrine), followed by the steroid cortisol. The heart speeds up and pumps harder, the nerves fire more quickly, the skin cools and gets goose bumps, the eyes dilate to see better, and the brain receives a message that it is time to do something.

We need to know when another animal is threatening to attack us in order to kill us and eat us. The fact that this particular threat doesn't exist anymore outside of the darkest jungles doesn't mean that fear can no longer be useful, as it is when we stand too close to the edge of a building or turn the wrong way down a one-way street. Triggers of fear involve sudden or dramatic changes in our environment, including dark, light, cold, heat, noise, isolation, or irritation. We react by getting ready, either to attack the source of our fear or to move away from it.

But not all danger is palpable or immediate. Many of the things that scare us aren't sudden, surprising, or matters of life or death. Fear has many guises. For every change of life there is a new set of concerns. For every milestone there is a transition, and fear and foreboding are normal aspects of making these transitions. They are the body's way of cautioning us that the change may or may not be for the better.

People enter puberty, graduate from high school, leave home to attend college, have sex for the first time, get married, give birth to a child, lose a parent, face serious illness, have surgery, lose a spouse, and finally, face their own death. In each case, fearfulness may accompany the life adjustment as a physiological warning to go slow. The fear reaction is normal and even protective, provided that it wears off after a while. The body needs time to adjust to new circumstances, after which it should return to a state of normal function.

Fear is a natural reaction to the unknown and is part of our built-in defense against a potentially hostile environment. We are afraid of suffering and pain, and we seek to avoid it at all costs.

WHAT HAS GONE AWRY?

In recent years the climate of fear has changed.

Statistically, the industrialized world has never been safer. Many of us are living longer and more uneventfully. Nevertheless, we live in fear of worst-case scenarios. Over the past century, armed with scientific and technological breakthroughs, we Americans have dramatically reduced our risk in virtually every area of life, resulting in life spans 60 percent longer in 2000 than in 1900. Antibiotics have reduced the likelihood of dying from infections. It used to be that a person could die from a scratch. Now we gobble down antibiotics at the first sign of trouble. Public health measures dictate standards for drinkable water and breathable air. Our garbage is removed quickly. We live temperature-controlled, disease-controlled lives.

And yet, we worry more than ever before. The natural dangers are no longer there, but the response mechanisms are still in place, and now they are turned on much of the time. We implode, turning our adaptive fear mechanism into a maladaptive panicked response.

We are bombarded with information. We live by TV sound bite, by Internet hyperbite and by unsourced tweet. Medical information has become agenda-driven, exaggerated by the media and disseminated on the Internet. The expectation of perfect health is perpetuated by these sources. Illness is no longer accepted as part of the natural order of things, and as consumers, we have become terrified of all disease, even though most of the time, doctors can diagnose an illness and offer either a cure or an effective treatment. Still, we continue to worry.

Our brains are not being infiltrated or provoked to panic by accident. The government has exploited its role as our official protector, from

Homeland Security to the CDC. Airport screeners and the FBI are suppos-edly the last line of defense between a terrorist or a disease and the citizens of western Ohio.

Every warning about a scary new disease, every report of terror-ist chatter, and every ultra-frail senior citizen becomes a justification for some government worker's job, from a research scientist all the way to the president himself. Government officials and politicians employ the media megaphone to promote the idea that they are keeping the populace safe. Unfortunately, there is no direct evidence to prove this. After a while the public becomes desensitized and can't tell a real alert from the latest hype. This was one of the reasons we were so unprepared for COVID-19. We had heard the warnings too many times before.

Of course, government officials couldn't grab the media megaphone if the media themselves didn't make it available. The mass media tend to magnify the latest health concern and broadcast it to millions. This has the effect of elevating an issue to a grand scale and provoking panic way out of proportion to the risks. The craze of the moment appears to be a threat to our personal safety until it runs its course through the media spotlight.

The authorities we used to look to in the community have been replaced by unfeeling conglomerates that thrive in a climate of uncertainty. The old leather-handed pharmacist, who suggested what type of condoms or deodorant to buy, has been replaced by the impersonality of a twenty-four-hour, neon-beaming chain store. Our old librarian, once more inter-ested in children even than books, has given way to software; how much reassurance can be found in an Internet search engine or a video on insta-gram?

WHY HAVE WE BECOME SO DEFENSELESS?

When Lyme disease, a troublesome bacteria transmitted to humans by the bite of a deer tick, was first being hyped twenty years ago, one of my most rational patients, a mathematics professor, was certain he had it every time he got a rash, even when he was living in Los Angeles, a city with zero deer.

"The chances of your having it are almost nonexistent," I assured him.

"Forget probabilities, I can just feel it," he said on more than one occa-sion.

Ten years later, with Lyme very much on the increase but out of the media spotlight, this patient—who by this time had moved to deer-ridden Connecticut—no longer had concerns about the now prevalent Lyme disease, but worried instead about bioterrorism. As well as he understood probabilities and equations, when he turned on the news at night or read his newspaper in the morning, he often personalized the latest risk and became worried that he might die.

With COVID, he burrowed away in his Connecticut bunker for months, not coming out even when the new case count in the state dropped very low. With no contact with anyone and no telltale symptoms, he felt certain he'd had it, even after negative COVID test and antibody results told him he hadn't.

Like my professor patient, we absorb the sense of urgency and believe we are in danger. So busy are we obsessing with one threat that we ignore the rest.

With over 8 million cases of tuberculosis every year in the world, 5 million new cases of AIDS, over 300 million cases of malaria, and over a million deaths due to each, Americans rarely worry about these diseases. In the United States approximately 40,000 people die of influenza every year, a statistic that went unnoticed until it was the flu's turn on the wheel of hype.

We brace ourselves for the next bug du jour and forgot all about the last one.

Many of the bugs du jour are cause for concern only among a certain segment of the population. Only a small portion of those who believe they are at risk really are, and few who become infected actually die. But a strange disease that kills only a few people still makes for good headlines if the story is strategically hyped. Many news teasers use the line "Are you and your family at risk?" The answer is usually no, but that tagline generates concern in every viewer, and this is what keeps people tuned in. If we didn't fundamentally misunderstand the risk, we probably wouldn't watch.

One year, during a flu vaccine shortage, I wrote an article in a local newspaper that the vaccine that year was only 40–60 percent effective, and was intended mostly for high-risk groups. My message: flu vaccine is not the health panacea that you think it is, you are not in great danger without it, and the sudden attention it is receiving has caused people to feel a sense of urgency out of proportion to the real danger.

I thought I'd accomplished something until I began to receive phone calls from patients who had read my piece. Almost as an afterthought I'd mentioned that I had five vials, or fifty doses, to give to my sickest patients.

"I saw your article," one call began.

"Are you reassured?" I asked.

The patient ignored me. "I understand you have some vaccine. Can I have a shot?"

Rather than worrying less after learning the facts, each patient wanted to be one of the lucky fifty and was calling me to beg for a dose.

Reeducating the public when it came to panic took far more than a corrective article that unintentionally became part of the hype.

When the media or the government focuses on a health scare, we all feel it, as though it's a palpable danger. When media attention is diverted elsewhere, the manifested fear fades but remains below the surface, waiting to attach itself to the next hyped target.

We are both controlled and divided through fear. Rather than enjoy the safety that our technological advances have provided us, instead we feel uncertain. Our personal fear alerts are turned on all the time. Fear is not intrinsically pathological, it is a reaction to the pathology of our times.

We feel the stress and have become more prone to irritability, disagreement, worry, insomnia, anxiety, and depression. We are more likely to experience chest pain, shortness of breath, dizziness, and headache.

We resist answers and torture ourselves with more and more questions. We ask—who can a frightened person count on for reliable information and reassurance?

MANAGING FEAR LIKE A DISEASE

Why are some people infected with hysteria out of proportion to the risks, while others seem impervious? Some of my patients worry over every symptom, while others never seem afraid of disease or death.

I recall a stoic ninety-three-year-old patient who had been a professional tap dancer for many years. She continued to dance in recitals despite her advancing age, until her back gave out. She went to several surgeons, all of whom advised against surgery, citing discouraging statistics. But she wasn't afraid. She had faith in her body and its ability to survive the surgery. Her passion for dancing outweighed any conceivable risk.

"Can the surgery help me dance again?" she asked me.

"It's possible."

"Then I'll take my chances," she said.

She sailed through the surgery and was dancing again a month later. For this patient, no matter how many times I warned her about potential risk, she replied that she believed she would be fine, and the cycle of worry never started.

Ultimately, we must develop prescriptions for the range of fears that patients' experience. These prescriptions must be practical and designed to break the cycle of worry. Those in society who inform us and who care for us—whether in government, the media, or health care—should be committed to maintaining a perspective based on realistic assessments of risk, rather than an agenda based on politics or profit.

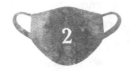

IT WORKS FOR ANIMALS BUT NOT FOR US

Take a rat and put it in a cage with a plexiglass divider.
It sees the cat on the other side. It's afraid it's going
to be attacked. The associated fear is very difficult
to extinguish, even with the plexiglass there.

—Esther Sabban, professor and graduate program director,
Department of Biochemistry and Molecular Biology, New York Medical College

When a patient is restrained inside a magnetic resonance imaging (MRI) machine during a scan of the brain, his head is strapped down and his body is enclosed in a coffinlike chamber. A loud metallic banging sound is heard, and the patient, like a restrained animal, may feel like he is never going to be released. The claustrophobia combines with the loud banging to cause an escalating fear.

Even worse is the terror some women feel when undergoing a mammogram. One of my patients described what it's like to wait while her breast has been painfully flattened to a pancake by the pressure of the equipment. "I have the awful fantasy," she said, "that the technician will die of a sudden heart attack or there will be a power outage, and my breast won't be released."

A patient's instinct is to fight her confinement, even when she knows it is for her own good. This is the same instinct an animal experiences. In fact, accepting ourselves as animals is crucial to understanding how human fear is designed to work. The fear center of the human brain, the amygdala, is identical to the primitive fear center of the animal brain.

Dr. Joseph Ledoux, a prominent neuroscientist and the author of The Emotional Brain, has studied fear extensively. He told me: "When a rat is afraid and when a human is afraid, very similar things occur in the body." But Ledoux also believes that triggers of fear vary dramatically from species to species. He said, "When a monkey is attacked, it will give off calls to other monkeys that something has happened. If a rat is under attack by a cat, it will give off an ultrasonic frequency in the range of rats, not cats. The frequency will be too high for a cat to hear."

Ledoux described the amygdala as "the hub in the brain's wheel of fear." When the amygdala is stimulated, there is an outpouring of stress hormones, causing a state of hypervigilance. The amygdala processes the primitive emotions of fear, hate, love, bravery, and anger—all neighbors in the deep limbic brain that we inherit from animals. When the amygdala malfunctions, a mood disorder, or state of uncontrollable apprehension, results.

The amygdala works together only with other brain centers that feed it and respond to it (the pre-frontal cortex). This fear hub senses via the thalamus (the brain's receiver), thinks through the cortex (the brain's seat of reasoning), and remembers via the hippocampus (the brain's file cabinet).

This cycle can become self-perpetuating. Here's an example of how it works: many years ago my young son was terrified by a sudden barking when we were hiking on a mountain trail at sunset.

I said, "The dog is gone," but he said, "No it's not. It keeps coming back."

For years afterward, each time a dog barked, it engaged the same mechanism. My son's thalamus triggered his amygdala, which retrieved the fearful memory for him from the hippocampus, and his body went into hyperdrive.

When the amygdala detects a threatening situation, out pour the stress hormones. The hippocampus alerts the amygdala's circuitry to a danger associated with a scary memory. At the same time, the hippocampus is also the center for caution. Under stress, the amygdala signals release while the hippocampus cautions slow down.

If the stress persists, the thinking brain falters, routine memories and behaviors shut down, and fear predominates. Previous trauma biases the brain toward fear pathways, which continue to fire again and again during flashbacks. This explains why even when we may not consciously remember a traumatic event, we retain a powerful emotional memory that we cannot reason ourselves away from. When the amygdala fires, it transmits fear signals too rapidly and powerfully for any of the brain's regular brakes to stop it.

Once a person has learned to fear something, he may always feel fear associated with that experience. But unlike mice, we humans can fear events we have only read or heard about, and so we worry about disasters we may never experience.

If we are unable to respond for lack of an appropriate target, the fear accumulates, and we become anxious.

FEAR CONDITIONING

Fear is user-ready at birth. As we grow, we are conditioned to respond to certain triggers. The fear response becomes automatic, though the dangers may not always be visible. If you put a rat in a box and shock it in the presence of a tone, it will become conditioned to respond to the shock, the tone, and the box. This contextual response helps an animal protect itself. The ability to recognize the box increases the likelihood of surviving the danger within by reacting quickly.

We are not rats, but we react similarly in terms of our primitive conditioning. Once a fear response is triggered, it may not diminish over time. Sometimes fears incubate, become indelible, and even increase in potency. They are often brought back to life by stressful events. This is both good and bad. It is useful for us to be able to remember situations associated with past dangers. But these memories may find their way into our daily lives, intruding on situations where the fears have no use, causing panic, phobias, or posttraumatic stress. We may feel compelled to avoid anything associated with a seminal fear event, including something that is neutral or even positive. If a barking dog bites a child, it may even lead to a self-defeating fear of all loud noises (including concert music), not just an adaptive fear of dogs.

The dangers that provoke the fear response in humans can be real or imagined, concrete or abstract. We may witness them firsthand or hear about them from others. We have a far greater capacity to imagine dangers than a rat does, and the potential for misperception is one of the major concerns of this book.

Drs. Robert and Caroline Blanchard have studied how humans evaluate situations for risk using our most highly evolved brain functions. Despite our advanced evolution, we often fail to assess the level of risk accurately. We humans tend to overpersonalize risk and to experience an unrealistic sense of danger whenever we hear or read of a bad event occurring to someone else. Many of my patients going for a routine CT scan will worry that they have a serious illness as soon as they see the sicker patients in the waiting room. My parents, healthy but in their mid nineties, respond with a "We'll be next" attitude whenever an ambulance is called to the retirement complex in Florida where they live.

A PRIMAL RESPONSE

Humans transmit danger signals in a way different from that used by animals. Ledoux said, "Social communication is greater for humans than for any other species. But it is difficult for humans to communicate fear accurately. The evolution of the human brain allows us to have ideas that don't match reality that well. This mismatch is a source of human anxiety."

All fear systems are intended to increase the likelihood of surviving a dangerous situation. Ledoux has shown that this response fires so rapidly and so powerfully that it overrides conscious thought.

A balding man in his fifties with intensely focused eyes and a resonant voice, Ledoux gave a careful reasoned talk on the neuroscience of fear at New School University on February 6, 2004, as part of a multidisciplinary conference there.

"Fear is a natural part of life," Ledoux said. "A snake on a path in the woods is threatening. So is an angry human. We respond with bodily upheaval. Fight or flight. Muscles tighten in response to a threat or in anticipation of one. We come into the world knowing how to be afraid. We learn what to be afraid of."

All animals with a backbone also have an amygdala. It takes only twelve milliseconds, according to Ledoux, for the thalamus to process sensory input and signal the amygdala. He called this emotional brain the "low road." The high road, or the thinking brain, takes thirty to forty milliseconds to process what is happening. The hippocampal memory center provides the context. "People have fear they don't understand or can't control because it is processed by the low road," Ledoux said.

The emotional brain also has its own intrinsic fear memory. Cells remember the fear and don't need to be reactivated, or reminded. Rats automatically respond to dangers they've seen previously.

During stress, reasoned memory is impaired, and emotional memory predominates, since the amygdala sends more signals to the thinking brain than the other way around. Humans are at the mercy of fear impulses that override reason. The upper brain tries to regulate fear, but its brakes are often ineffective at slowing the powerful emotions of the system. Valium and Prozac block the amygdala by different mechanisms, creating an artificial shield against fear.

Take away the amygdala and you take away fear. In 1999 researchers at the University of Southern California and the Université de Bordeaux published a study in Nature in which they demonstrated the role of the amygdala in emotional memory. They implanted electrodes in the brains of laboratory mice and measured the strong response to a tone and a subsequent electric shock. When the amygdala was surgically removed, both the animals' panicked immobility and the frenetic brain wave pattern disappeared.

Similar results have been found in humans who have suffered trauma and damage to the amygdala. They become unable to feel afraid even when they are presented with clear danger signals.

At that fear conference sixteen years ago, Ledoux spoke about the nature of the fear response across the entire animal kingdom. "Fear is learned instantly. Fear is remembered forever. Fear is self-sustaining. Fear motivates other kinds of behavior that are designed to affect its impact."

But inevitably, an appropriate fear response depends on access to accurate information. As Ledoux said, "Will fear be based on an honest assessment of the threat, or will it be trumped up?"

CHARACTERISTICS OF FEAR

Back in the mid-1980s, Isaac Marks, a prominent fear theorist, described the basic fear responses of withdrawal, immobility, fighting back, or submission. When these responses are not effective or when they become internalized over a period of time, anxiety may well result.

What distinguishes fear reactions between humans and other animals is not the physiology of fear but the triggers that activate it. For humans, our added brainpower allows defensive reactions to more and more triggers. Hence, we are more prone to social anxiety.

Fear also has a genetic component. A rat will rev up in response to the odor of a fox even if that rat has spent its whole life in the laboratory. Humans are automatically fearful of situations that threatened our ancestors.

FEAR PATHOLOGY

Arne Ohman, a leader in the field of human fear and anxiety, has argued that panic, phobia, and posttraumatic stress all emanate from unremitting fears.

In his landmark book, *The Emotional Brain,* Ledoux showed how pathological anxiety evolves from the basic mechanisms of fear. Anxiety manifests itself in different ways: Phobias are avoidance fears that can't be suppressed, panic attacks are circumscribed periods of intense anxiety, and free-floating anxiety is worry that goes on and on. Obsessive-compulsive disorder involves rituals that are intended to neutralize anxiety but end up enhancing it by being so excessive. With posttraumatic stress disorder (PTSD), the fear response fails to diminish with the passage of time.

Psychotherapy is an attempt to retrain the higher centers of the brain to exert control over the lower centers, including the amygdala. This approach is similar to trying to rein in an untamed stallion. The amygdala may rear up at any time.

POSTTRAUMATIC STRESS

Dr. Rachel Yehuda, a professor of psychiatry at Mount Sinai School of Medicine, is a passionate researcher and a pioneer in understanding posttraumatic stress disorder. Her findings suggest that it is cortisol that helps the body adapt to heavy trauma over time. Without this crucial steroid to aid in coping, a trauma victim can fall into a pattern of unremitting fear.

In Dr. Yehuda's experience, many people exposed to extreme trauma do not develop PTSD precisely because cortisol protects them. She described

PTSD to me in an interview as "a failure to control the adaptive mechanism of the fear response." The key to a perpetual state of terror, according to Yehuda, is an inability to suppress the amygdala. "The usual limbic brake on the amygdala isn't working. Cortisol is supposed to initiate this. Without it, the stress response isn't contained."

The popularizing of PTSD in the media has led many who aren't truly terrorized to use it as an excuse for their hysteria. Overstatement dilutes the language of terror and renders it less useful. "The mention of posttraumatic stress occurs when there is a shortage of terms for laypeople to use for their vulnerabilities when confronted by trauma," said Yehuda.

People who are afraid to get on a bus because they have seen a suicide bombing on the news are overpersonalizing a danger. This isn't really PTSD. It is an inflated perception of risk. Yehuda said, "In America, we worry about whether something that hasn't happened could happen. In Israel, when something does happen, we worry about it occurring again."

HOW HUMANS LEARN TO FEAR

We humans take for granted that language helps us to negotiate our world, but it is also true that we often misuse and misinterpret words. The fear response works best based on nonverbal cues. When we humans try to use abstract language to communicate threats, we too easily overload and provoke the fear response.

Dr. Elizabeth Phelps, a psychologist and neuroscientist now at Harvard University, has examined how our brains respond to threats we only envision. Although people learn about dangerous events through hard experience—a dog is deemed dangerous because it once bit you—we also learn about dangers by watching—you observe a dog bite someone else.

Using highly sensitive MRI scans, Phelps discovered that the amygdala can be activated in response to dangers a person merely observes. Phelps concluded that fear activation based on watching is just as powerful as direct experience, but easily prone to misinterpretation. She said to me, "When you are watching it and you are told that it is going to happen to you, it causes the same robust response by the amygdala as if you experienced it yourself."

TURNING OFF FEAR

In November 2002 researchers working for the National Institute of Mental Health published a study in Nature that described a way to turn off fear. Stimulating the front part of a rat's brain with an electrode caused it to automatically emit a "safety signal" that signaled the amygdala to slow down. When a tone was repeatedly presented to rats without the loud "danger" tone that at first accompanied it, over time the safety signal caused them to become less and less afraid.

In December 2002 researchers at Columbia University discovered the gene that turns off fear in mice. The results were reported in the journal *Cell*.

In September 2004 Dr. Phelps used specialized MRI to study the human brain, and she discovered fear extinction circuits in humans that correspond to those previously identified in rats. Phelps recognized the limitations of the animal model but concluded that our cognitive mechanisms are "interacting with the same circuitry as animals have."

Like rats, humans can temporarily turn off fear, though in both cases the wiring heavily favors the on switch. Unlike rats, we humans are forever trying to turn off something that should never have been turned on in the first place. "Extinction is not erasing a fear but trying to control it," Phelps said to me.

OUR CONSTANT STATE OF ALERT

Dr. Esther Sabban has studied fear by restraining animals. She believes the animals react to the loss of control and "not knowing if it's ever going to end." Dr. Sabban's work shows that animals that have been exposed to one danger have an exaggerated response to a new danger. When she exposed an animal to the cold, the animal could become used to it and learn not to react. But the same animal was then hypersensitive to being restrained. The fear neurochemicals shot up higher and stayed that way for many days after the animal was untied. In other words, certain primitive fears can't be extinguished even when there is no danger.

Once fear has been activated, it can lead to overreactions in all directions. This is how we feel when we are told that we could be attacked again by an unseen force like al-Qaeda. The fear response may well be suppressed over time, but it can resurface—stronger than before—and even extend to all aspects of our lives. A person who thinks he has gotten used to the orange terror alert message on the TV screen may nevertheless experience a hyperalert response seeing someone with a gun in an airport, even if that person is a security guard. This new state of hyperalertness originates in neurochemical fear memory that develops over time. The capacity for desensitization is limited because the amygdala is stronger. It takes a lot of psychotherapy to override the fear message, and the fear center wakes up again with each new stimulus that comes along.

It is worrisome to consider what this state of free-floating communicated fear does to our bodies. We gain or lose weight, our immune systems become overloaded, and we become susceptible to diseases that we might otherwise have been able to resist.

WHAT WE GET FROM APES

Apes, like humans, have highly developed brain centers, with sophisticated memory and some ability to reason. But unlike humans, other primates appear to have a dependable society that determines what alarms them. I spoke with Dr. Chris Jolly, a good-natured British anthropologist at New York University, who maintains that apes have honest fear responses. Jolly has investigated aggressive behavior among baboons.

"Are threats among primates always real?" I asked him.

"Usually," he said, "primates don't use referential communication. Warning signals concern things that are directly dangerous. They don't use fear talk to distract."

I considered danger as perceived by the animal world. Has our technology made us too smart for our own good? Even if the animal world is more dangerous than ours, it is more honest: the threat of attack—when it occurs—is real.

"All animals that live in societies have a pecking order," Jolly said, "including chickens, where the expression comes from. Part of organizing into an animal society is to decide who is more powerful than you—animals convey a submissive posture to others who are dominant to them. In more intelligent mammals, like wolves, for example, fear is based on a memory of what the enemy has done in the past. There is a structure of tensions, flux in the hierarchy, young animals coming up to replace the older ones going down. The adherence to the structure provides comfort."

"We humans have created environments that don't comfort us," I said, and Dr. Jolly laughed.

"Can the same thing happen to other primates?" I asked. "Can they lose touch with real threats and create pseudothreats like humans do?"

Jolly paused, thinking carefully about this before he spoke.

"Rhesus monkeys have been studied in captivity. When they're crammed into smaller spaces like the animal equivalent of cities, they become more aggressive and more fearful. They also experience more stress and fear in ambiguous situations and in situations of change."

"This is true for humans as well."

Jolly agreed that in certain crowded baboon and chimpanzee societies we begin to see the fear-provoking abstractions that are so prevalent among us humans.

Dr. Robert Sapolsky, a researcher at Stanford, has examined baboon behavior under stress. By measuring stress hormones found in their stool, Sapolsky was able to determine that baboons, like humans, live in high-stress societies, with order maintained by intimidation. Sapolsky also showed that living in fear damages a baboon's health and, as with humans, that sustained production of stress hormones can damage the hippocampus, affecting learning and memory.

Chimps are probably the only nonhuman primate with a sense of self. "They can put themselves in the position of other chimps," Jolly said. "Chimps fool each other. They use deceptive behavior to get gain."

"This deception causes other chimps to be afraid of them?"

"The same as with humans," Jolly said.

Dr. Jane Goodall has studied chimpanzees extensively. Pertaining to fear, she observed that a band of young male chimps tenses up when it approaches the border of their group's domain, psyching themselves up for the possibility of battle with neighboring chimp groups, a form of danger recognition. When the chimps menace each other purely for the sake of control or domination, they are exhibiting traits recognizable in their self-defeating human counterparts.

WHAT WE GET FROM EACH OTHER

Dr. Paul Ekman has studied danger recognition in humans. In his book *Emotions Revealed*, he wrote that we can learn to be afraid of anything.

Ekman focused on the facial expressions we use to communicate worry to each other. Worry about an impending threat causes muscular tension. Ekman observed that raised upper eyelids are fundamental in communicating fear. Unfortunately, these expressions can't easily communicate the degree of the threat, which is why expressions of fear are infectious and may alarm others unnecessarily.

Like rats, we have defined pathways for invoking fear and for attempting to suppress or extinguish it. Like rats, when we are caught in a maze of fear, we may learn to navigate for a time, but the price is a state of hyper-alert vigilance that burns up our metabolism and renders us more susceptible to illness.

In addition to the fight-or-flight conditioned fear that we inherit from animals, there are the elaborate communicated and learned fear and worry that we humans alone possess and that we inflict on each other. The anticipation of danger based on risk involves the brain's highest centers, which then connect to the amygdala and cause the reverberating states of panic and worry.

This human fear is not reasonable but is driven by fragmented information, hype, miscommunication, and uncertainty. If we are unable to convert our uncertainty into a reasoned assessment of risk, we grow more and more afraid, caught up in a cycle of worry. Feeling safe means coming to realize that the probability of harm occurring to us is very small.

Feeling safe also means returning fear to its proper place as an animal instinct. Reason and abstract thinking are human trademarks. Our language is ill suited to communicating primitive emotions. Perhaps we can learn from animals a more limited but appropriate use of fear.

OUR CULTURE
OF WORRY

What an appalling affront to share the intense desire
for continued existence with all living things
but be smart enough to recognize the ultimate futility
of this most basic biological imperative.
We think that clash creates the potential for terror.

—Tom Pyszczynski, professor of psychology at the University of Colorado
and cofounder of terror management theory

Animals may fear death as much as we do, but whereas animals freeze in the face of immediate danger, we experience an ongoing existential fear, connected to our unique self-awareness. Our central fear of death reaches beyond our animal instincts and may threaten to overwhelm us. But like all our fears, our fear of death is overblown when we are wrongly convinced that death is in the offing. Our fear of death is so pervasive it is too easily provoked.

At the New School University fear conference back in 2004, Dr. Tom Pyszczynski, a rumple-jacketed professor with flowing white hair, was a striking contrast to the balding, impeccably dressed Ledoux. Pyszczynski was one of the originators of terror management theory, and he described how all fear emanates from a primary fear of death. "Fear is supposed to function to keep us alive and help us stave off death. As an unpleasant emotion, it creates a barrier we're not supposed to cross."

Dr. John Mann, currently a professor of translational neuroscience at Columbia University and the director of molecular imaging and neuropathology at the New York State Psychiatric Institute, is an expert on suicide. In an interview, he said that even in the most extreme cases, fear of death is designed to have a protective aspect. "Take away this fear inhibition, and the person is no longer indecisive, and suicide may ensue."

But even if fear can be protective, it can also be destructive. As the only species that is aware of the inevitability of death, we have a great need for our culture to give us a sense of meaning and purpose. The growing unease in our society is testament to the fact that our culture is no longer capable of doing the job. Pyszczynski theorized that fear out of control erodes our perceived wellness. This fear of death, while essential, is self-defeating if it paralyzes people.

In order to buffer our dread, humans try to construct a shield—a value-laden belief system that bolsters our self-esteem and allows us to sublimate our greatest fears. We attempt to manage terror through a complex psychological defense mechanism. Our primary instinct to circumvent death becomes our drive to make art, pursue science, and construct civilizations that are intended to last beyond our years. The drive to have children is a biological, as well as a cultural, answer to the fear of death. Overall, we feel safer when we participate in this culture.

Unfortunately, this instinct toward culture may easily be transformed into a negative culture of worry. Multiple studies in the psychiatric literature over the past few decades have corroborated the link between fear of death and thinking negatively about others. The culture of fear is one that breeds prejudice and distrust.

The growing epidemic of fear also encourages the expectation of illness and death. Many of us are overly afraid of illnesses we don't have. We may personalize the risk of death while lacking any disease that could cause death. And once we have an illness, many fear an outcome much more ominous than the one indicated by reliable medical data.

Cancer used to serve as a graphic illustration of this phenomenon. While the public advocacy campaign for cancer prevention shone a necessary light on the evils of cigarette smoking and carcinogens, it also made people more fearful. Cancer is still described too often in value-laden terminology like "end stage" or "pervasive." This has started to change over the last few years thanks to immunotherapy and biotechnology. Unfortunately, there is still a shock related to a cancer diagnosis and for many, it is still assumed to be a death sentence. Thanks to technology, diagnoses are made quickly. One day you think you are healthy, the next you have a life-threatening illness. Therapies are now perceived as evolving and state-of-the-art which has helped with the anti-fear messaging.

In the late 1990s, HIV/AIDS fell out of the U.S. health care news cycle and stopped scaring us, and now finally the reality has begun to catch up with the news, as less than a 800,000 people died of HIV/AIDS worldwide in 2018. Global health efforts, including the President's Emergency Plan for AIDS Relief (PEPFAR), launched by President George W. Bush in 2003, have helped, though there is a long way to go, many millions are living successfully with HIV.

But cancer continues to scare us, in part because we can't seem to control when and if we get it. Most patients are even frightened of the screening tests such as mammograms and colonoscopies that make it possible to treat cancer before it can kill them. Once cancer is found, and even if it is cured, fear is the uninvited guest that whispers of its possible recurrence even with the latest treatments. As threatening as a cancer is, fear of death from cancer's insidious tentacles is even worse.

The culture of cancer care does its best to alleviate these fears. Chemotherapy and immunotherapy involve multiple social workers and self-help support groups which are frequently represented on-line The radiation suite at our hospital is a calm therapeutic milieu, including an aquarium with an extensive collection of multicolored tropical fish.

Unfortunately, the culture of hyped fears offsets many of these attempts at support and insight. Fueled by fragments of bad news from media, Internet, and Social Media sources, patients still fear the worst-case scenario—a painful imminent death.

ONE PATIENT'S FEAR OF DEATH

My waiting room was filled with patients, but one in particular was telling the nurse that he couldn't bear to wait another moment. He was peering at her through tiny spectacles, better suited for a much older patient, which had slid to the end of his nose.

He was a forty-four-year-old international businessman, and I could hear his nervous accented speech through the waiting room window glass.

I'd ordered a CT scan on "Ephraim Azziz" because he was a smoker. I reassure smokers that the test is routine, that I am being compulsive, that a

CT scan is more sophisticated than an X-ray in analyzing a smoker's lungs. But almost all smokers fear cancer, and it takes a negative result to truly reassure them. Knowing that a CT scan or other state-of-the-art test can foretell their future puts many patients in a state of worry as soon as they are told to have the scan.

Azziz went for the scan a few weeks after seeing me. The report came to me a few days later, indicating a three-centimeter nodule at the top of the right lung, consistent with cancer. Upon seeing the report, I told the office nurse that I needed to see Ephraim Azziz right away.

By the time I saw him in the examination room, he was as nervous as I ever remember seeing a patient. He appeared ultrathin, gray around his temples, with piercing eyes.

"The report says there's a nodule there," I said. "We have to biopsy it. But it's small. And there are no swollen lymph nodes. It may well not be cancer. If it is, worst-case scenario, we should be able to operate on it and cure you."

"I want to know as soon as possible," he said, squeezing his ears and scratching the sides of his face, a gesture that conveyed extreme nervousness. He squirmed on the examination table. I performed a limited examination, as I'd just seen him a few weeks before. I invited him into my corner consultation room, a sanctum with walls of white brick and many windows. Mr. Azziz seemed to relax somewhat as he sank into the soft leather chair, as if the news couldn't get any worse in here.

I decided to show the CT scan to my office mate at the time, "Dr. Madison." A prominent pulmonologist, he didn't accept Mr. Azziz's insurance, but he was always willing to give me his opinion on an X-ray or CT scan.

He crisply snapped the scan up onto his view box. This type of doctorly precision and familiarity with potential cancers could frighten a patient if he saw it. The report already had the words "SUSPICIOUS FOR A BRONCHOGENIC NEOPLASM" written on it. The radiologist had pronounced sentence on a man he'd never met. Such an anonymous practice helps provoke patient panic.

A great diagnostician and a feeling physician, my office partner always looked for nuances. He analyzed all the possibilities, reluctant to jump to a conclusion at this stage. "It could be cancer," Madison said. "But it might just be scar. Needs a biopsy, but it could well be negative."

I brought this happy news right back to Azziz, and I could see a visible change. He stopped moving his hands back and forth in a purposeless pattern, and now he wiped his sweaty forehead with the back of his sleeve. Madison had introduced a tangible hope. We could envision a scenario that didn't involve cancer or require surgery. Cancer gave mortality a name and a timetable, but a negative result would return mortality to the abstract.

Still, as he rose to go, I could almost feel the animal fear welling up like an unstoppable current that would not ebb.

We both pressed to know the answer as soon as we could. Pushing hard past impassive clerks and loaded appointment schedules and the antagonistic world of low quality insurance coverage, I gave this man all the priority and VIP status I could muster, internally with my staff and externally with other staffs. I could sense his helplessness, his guilt over his years of smoking, putting his three children at risk of a fatherless future.

He was overwhelmed by the mushrooming fear of his illness. He was under the control of this fear, and he could only hope to defeat it with the knowledge that the cancer wasn't there, couldn't be there, because the tissue itself said it wasn't true.

The degree of his worry was tied to imagining what he might feel if the cancer was there. Even if the surgery cured it and he faced only the specter of the cancer's returning, the fear would recur first. In Azziz's case, fear would be much more difficult to control than cancer. If there was a positive aspect to this fear, it was that Azziz would be too frightened to ever smoke again.

Azziz was lucky in one respect—medical testing would lead to a definite answer. Many times the patient is kept in limbo; for example, an MRI of the brain might show some signal abnormalities that could indicate multiple sclerosis. What is a doctor supposed to tell a patient who goes for an MRI because of a headache and comes back with a result that could mean she has this stigmatizing, disabling disease? Sometimes the technology increases the uncertainty. Some patients have to live under the shroud of worry that comes with a possible diagnosis.

For Azziz, at least, a definitive answer would be forthcoming, though now that his illusion of health had been disrupted, his worry was bound to persist.

Two weeks later, when he returned to my office, I was amazed to discover that he still hadn't had the biopsy. He'd found a pulmonologist who accepted his insurance, and this doctor had suggested a PET scan first to sense activity in the nodule before doing the biopsy. He'd also done a skin test for tuberculosis that turned out to be positive. Apparently the lung doctor, "Dr. Saby," had said the nodule could be a scar from tuberculosis rather than cancer. This was potentially good news, but Azziz seemed too worried to consider it. Azziz was picking up stray comments from his growing ensemble of doctors, and he was trying to put them together in some kind of order that would predict his future.

Instead of being reassured, he was more confused and frightened. He stuck out his arm and pointed to the cherry-red spot in the center, which was the positive skin test for TB. "Do I have TB too?" he asked. "Should I be treated for it? Wear a mask?"

We bypassed the examination room—I decided he had had enough examinations for the time being—and sat in my consultation room. He leaned forward on the couch across from me. Each new piece of information made him question how all the pieces fit together. In order to gain that elusive perspective as he obsessed over the potentially devastating illness, he had to hear the facts in a certain order, like the combination to a vault.

Dr. Saby, by being thorough and careful, had unintentionally alarmed Azziz further. Each new sophisticated test created another reason to worry, and delay only allowed the patient's fear to grow.

"You do not have active tuberculosis," I said.

Azziz smiled, glad there was something he didn't have.

A week later, my assistant placed the PET scan report on my desk with a message to call Azziz. I hesitated, not wanting to convey results via the telephone. Personal contact between doctor and patient helps a patient to put news in perspective instead of panicking. The more impersonal the communication, the more fear is transmitted along with the message.

But sometimes if I request a face-to-face discussion, the patient immediately assumes the worst. This approach had already backfired with Azziz. Some patients prefer to communicate by e-mail, but e-mail is not the place for serious results. I decided to try the telephone this time.

"Mr. Azziz, I have the results of your PET scan. The area of the nodule is a hot area."

"What does this mean?"

"It means it's not a scar. Something's going on there."

"What could it be?"

"It could be a tumor. But it's very small. It can be removed," I said.

Silence.

Without the help of facial expressions and a calm demeanor, it was difficult for me to convey the concept of "curable" and have it outweigh the concept of "tumor." I found I couldn't alleviate his nervousness over the phone as well as I could in person.

"I can't sleep," he said.

"Would you like a sleeping pill?"

"Okay," he said, sighing. "I'm going for the needle biopsy Thursday." There were no tests left to delay the biopsy, no more doctors to see.

The next time I heard from him was when he called from the waiting room before his biopsy.

"I've waited three hours already, and the doctor isn't here, but his partner showed up and wanted to do the biopsy. I sent him away. What should I do? Should I go home?"

I urged Azziz to let the second doctor do the procedure. His ambivalence about who performed it seemed another manifestation of his worry. He was trying to control his fear by creating more choices for himself.

He later described the radiologist as unsmiling behind a paper mask and gown. Mr. Azziz said he felt at the time that the doctor's unsympathetic posture was another indication that a cancer diagnosis was in the offing.

Rather than allowing the patient to succumb to premonitions or speculations that stoke the amygdala, it is important for a physician to have a strategy for dealing with the specter of cancer. This strategy must be based on a reasoned assessment of the facts, since most patients become more frightened if they think you are deceiving them.

"Dr. Yang," the cytologist (an expert in cells), called me with the results two days after the biopsy was taken. It was two hours before the start of Yom Kippur, the Jewish day of atonement. "It's squamous cell carcinoma of the lung," he said.

Squamous cancer meant skin cells in the lung gone berserk.

There was no good way to deliver bad news. I wondered if Azziz, who was religious, might have preferred to know his fate as he prayed for forgiveness on Yom Kippur. Still, I decided to wait to tell him until after the holiday so that I could have a plan in place when I spoke with him.

On Tuesday, when Azziz leaned across from me in my consultation room, he seemed strangely detached, rather than expectant.

"I have the results," I began. "You do have a small cancer, but it's contained, it hasn't spread, it's curable by surgery."

"I know," he replied. "Dr. Saby called me with the results this morning."

"Saby?"

"Said he recommended surgery. Said he was happy that the tumor hadn't spread. Said I should go for chemotherapy afterwards just as an insurance policy."

Saby had charged to center stage before I could get there. He was the head of our hospital's end-of-life team, and he was used to facing cancer. He was a bullish doctor, but he was also highly skilled and responsible.

"Knowing made me feel better," Azziz said. "Imagining was far worse than knowing."

The knowledge that your future lies in a computerized scan or a tissue result can cause a welling up of uncontrollable panic. But when the definitive answer comes, the mystery is gone, which is for some the worst part. Unfortunately, fear of death remains a primary focus even in cancer that can be cured by surgery.

Azziz had come to this office visit with multiple printouts, charts, and information from various lung cancer Web sites. He knew the exact survival statistics and the worst-case scenario for his particular pathology. He was fully plugged in to our contemporary culture of worry.

"How do I know it won't come back?" he said, already seeing past the surgery to his future worry.

"This is squamous cell. A skin type that's also found in the lung. It tends to stay local and not spread."

I drew a picture of the lungs and showed his lesion perched atop the right lung, which had three lobes, whereas the left had only two. I told him that after the right upper lobe was removed, the remaining two lobes would expand over several months, and he would get almost all of his lung capacity back. I felt like a dry textbook, but he nodded slowly, contemplating, seeming partly reassured by the factoids and by the picture.

"Will I always need monitoring?"

"We'll continue to scan you, every six months at first, and then every year."

Azziz told me he'd rather not go to my hospital for his surgery, because of his miserable three-hour wait for the needle biopsy. I was unable to convince him that the inconvenience and confusion could happen anywhere, in any hospital. The most important things about the biopsy were that they'd gotten a good sample, the pathology had come back quickly, and the scans had shown limited disease.

"But it was chaos there," he said. "Some people were hanging out while others were mourning. People in wheelchairs and stretchers were in the hallways, and around them staff were laughing and joking. I didn't feel confident they would really send you my results and not mix them up with someone else's."

But Azziz was not reasoning out the role the hospital had actually played in sussing out his cancer. Disarray and disorganization make patients more fearful. He was attributing to my hospital a greater threat potential than I believed it had. This was all tied in with his emotional response to the news. His fear was deep and primitive, already verging on fight or flight. He couldn't reason through the actual risks presented by his cancer. He was consumed by the fear of death that cancer brings to many patients.

What stayed in Azziz's mind even after the good news of no spread was the threat of danger rather than the hope for cure. He remained on the alert. His fear wouldn't shut off. Instead of focusing on how to get better, he continued to collect information about how he might get worse, drawn from an interwoven network of alarming facts disseminated by the media.

I accepted his choice to leave my medical center. Just as allowing a trapped animal to choose a possible path of escape may diminish its terror, so with humans regaining control in life-or-death situations is a way to channel primitive fear.

Azziz was going to go uptown to the Memorial Sloan-Kettering Cancer Center. He would have his surgery and his chemotherapy there. Reputation didn't ensure outcome, but it made Azziz feel slightly more comfortable.

We would keep in touch by phone, and he would return to see me two weeks after the surgery. We shook hands and hugged before he left.

A HEALTHY PATIENT'S WORRY

As soon as Azziz left the office, I encountered another worried patient. "Nelly Foster" had been my patient for eight years, and I rarely treated her for anything beyond the muscle soreness that came from running the New York City marathon.

Occasionally, she would call me for bronchitis, and I would prescribe an antibiotic. Like many American doctors, I sometimes tend to over-prescribe antibiotics because of a placebo effect. There could be bacteria behind the coughing, but antibiotics also have a calming influence. Many patients are relieved by the doctor's taking action on their behalf.

Nelly was a patient who could not effectively use reason to diminish her fears. Nor did her extensive physical exercise routine help alleviate her concerns as it did for so many other patients. For Nelly, her worries required frequent attention and were out of proportion to the real risk of physical disease. She usually responded to large doses of my reassurance in addition to the occasional antibiotic.

This time, Nelly Foster was in a panic. She had been in to see me once weekly for the past three weeks. On the first visit she said she was so overcome with coughing and heavy breathing at night that she was petrified she might stop breathing altogether.

I'd diagnosed seasonal allergy plus a sinus infection, but antihistamines, antibiotics, steam, and a humidifier hadn't done the trick. On the second visit I prescribed a decongestant and a steroid nasal spray and arranged for her to see an allergist. Now she was back again, still overcome with worry, shouting at me in the examination room that the allergist had done nothing and that the only thing that helped her was the Robitussin the pharmacist had wisely offered.

But there was a greater agenda for Nelly Foster. She was getting married the following week, at the age of forty-seven, for the first time, to a man named Earl. Over the years that I'd taken care of her, she'd shared with me her desire to become pregnant even as her menstrual cycle waned. By the time she met Earl it was almost too late, and he, a veteran of one childless marriage already, said he didn't think he wanted children.

I mark my life by the milestones in my patients' lives, and now Nelly was coming to see me, not with child news, but with marriage news. A small ceremony was set for the following week, and I suddenly realized that Nelly's upcoming wedding had evoked feelings of grief over being childless. This marriage meant leaving behind for good her dream of having children.

When she acknowledged her commitment to Earl, she added that she was starting to feel better physically. She no longer felt like she would stop breathing in the middle of the night.

As much as treating her congestion, I realized I was performing a ritual of medical clearance for the next phase in her life. Each milestone is a marker on the road to a patient's death. For Nelly, these fears between milestones manifested themselves as nervous complaints.

No matter what a doctor does to counter the primary fear of illness and death, unmitigated fear can still take root. Uncertainty over illness is directly connected to a patient's fear of death. We humans have an instinctive fear of death, to which we add an awareness of death that easily overwhelms our ability to assess risk. Because of the power of this awareness, it is helpful if we can learn not to be afraid of diseases that don't directly threaten us.

FEAR BECOMES THE RISK

My nurse informed me that there was a new patient in my examination room. His name was "Donald Tribune," and he said he was the owner of a taxi company.

He had a raspy voice from many years of smoking three packs a day. He had been avoiding doctors for the past five years since an internist handed him a CT scan report of his lungs that mentioned the possibility of cancer but also read, "No discernible mass." Instead of repeating the scan in a few months the way the doctor had suggested, Tribune ran away, keeping the report in a back pocket and worrying that he was going to die at any time.

Tribune also kept a list of medications he was supposed to take but never did. As opposed to Nelly Foster, who was comforted by pills, for Tribune, medicines were reminders that good health was just an illusion.

Tribune sat in my consultation room right where Azziz had sat and began to weep when I told him that he might not have cancer. For five years he had lived with the fear while continuing to smoke at the same time. The X-ray taken in my office, like the previous CT scan, showed the scars of the smoke but no discernible mass.

We developed a rapport, and he decided to go for a new CT scan. The results came back a week later and confirmed no cancer.

DEATH BY FEAR

The end of this story is not a happy one. When fear becomes its own malignant disease, it can be as difficult to contain as any aggressive virus or tissue-transforming tumor.

Mr. Tribune remained so nervous despite his good news that his blood pressure rose. The original CT scan had primed his fear pump and kept him feeling chronically on the verge of catastrophe. He was anxious most of the time but wouldn't take medicine for anxiety, and he wouldn't see a psychotherapist. Finally, on one of his most anxious days, his blood pressure rose out of control—and with no one there to help him, he experienced a sudden bleed into his head and died.

PLAYING POLITICS WITH FEAR: POST 9/11

Bush, it's now clear, intends to run a campaign
based on fear. And for me, at least, it's working:
Thinking about what these people will do if they solidify
their grip on power makes me very, very afraid.

—Paul Krugman, New York Times, September 3, 2004

Our post-9/11 fears became a free-floating anxiety that lacked a specific target. We lacked information as to where, when, or how, or even whether, the threat was greater today than it was yesterday. We no longer know who to blame or who to follow to safety.

The collateral damage of these fears appeared to be many Americans' health. We were on perpetual alert status, which stoked safety concerns. This process wore us down and interfered with our ability to function.

MEET THE PRESS

On February 7, 2004, George W. Bush sat in the Oval Office and was interviewed by Tim Russert for NBC's Meet the Press. A major topic of discussion, amidst flagging public sentiment that the war in Iraq was necessary in order to somehow defend our national security, was President Bush's continuing assertion that Saddam Hussein had possessed weapons of mass destruction along with the ability to use them against us. During the interview, the president said, "Saddam Hussein was dangerous with weapons. He was a dangerous man in the dangerous part of the world."

There was certainly a worldwide consensus that Hussein was heinous. There was little argument with the fact that he'd authorized torture and brutal killing of multitudes in his region. But was he a direct threat to America?

Bush's rhetoric was intended to instill the notion that Hussein was the embodiment of the evil our country faced, and that Bush, our president, our protector, was the strong leader who had rid the world of the threat before its capacity to destroy us was realized. Bush said, "These are people who kill in a moment's notice. . . . When we see a threat we deal with a threat because they become imminent. . . . Saddam Hussein was a danger to America. . . . As president of the United States, my most solemn responsibility is to keep this country safe."

How many people tried to envision what was actually being suggested here—Saddam supplying the terrorists with a large stash of chemical or biological weapons that would be smuggled here undetected, culminating in a drone plane flying from offshore to deliver its payload unobserved, with the wind blowing in just the right direction?

But in reality chemical and biological weapons are effective WMDs only in an extreme worst-case scenario. Under most circumstances they would actually be WSDs, weapons of some destruction, still hardly comforting, but a more accurate term.

Nevertheless, the rhetoric of protection continued. As Bush said on Meet the Press, "The war against terrorists is a war against individuals who hide in caves in remote parts of the world, individuals who have these kind of shadowy networks, individuals who deal with rogue nations."

Notice how the terrorist description merged with the description of Saddam and his henchmen. If the public believed there was a single danger, embodied in Iraq and its tentacles, then the president would have been justified in sending our troops over there to protect us. In taking this strong stand, he was echoing the position taken by prior presidents, specifically Abraham Lincoln and Franklin Roosevelt, who were reelected based on a promise to protect us from dangers.

To continue selling the war, the Bush administration, like both Democrats and Republicans before it, kept generating fear.

The same kind of fearmongering was used in the overall fight against terror. As the years elapsed since September 11, 2001, bin Laden and his al-Qaeda network remained a primary justification for an elaborate world war on terror.

The ultimate argument was put forth by Harvard professor Michael Ignatieff in his book *The Lesser Evil.* Unless we extinguished these terrorists now, the argument went, they could mushroom into nuclear-weapon-wielding menaces who could blow up our cities. Wasn't it a small price to give up some liberties now rather than face an ineradicable danger later on?

The answer to this was no, if one believed that we couldn't allow fear to control us. Despite terrorism, the risk to the individual remained quite low.

Since it is difficult to actually quantify the real risk of a disaster, it is easy for politicians to motivate the public based on fear of the unknown or these worst-case scenarios. Time after time, the far-reaching fear and an increased sense of vulnerability tied to the World Trade Center attack were utilized by Bush and others in a public cry to protect us. Time after time, coached by our leaders, we personalized risks that were remote.

OUR PROTECTORS FROM WHAT?

While drawing our attention to these unlikely dangers, at the same time the government revealed a porous safety net, which spread more fear. As Robert Reich wrote harshly in the American Prospect in August 2004, "America's intelligence system failed to see terrorist threats coming from al-Qaeda prior to September 11 that should have been evident, and then, after 9/11, saw terrorist threats coming from Iraq that didn't exist. A system that doesn't warn of real threats and does warn of unreal ones is broken."

The Bush administration didn't properly police and regulate certain potential targets such as chemical plants . A 2002 Brookings Institution study, as well as a Government Accountability Office report, identified security at chemical plants as being underaddressed. The Brookings report held that chemical plants were not "adequately protected against terrorist attack." The GAO warned in March 2003 that "no one has comprehensively assessed the security of chemical facilities." Meanwhile, administration lawyers blocked efforts by the EPA to beef up security at chemical plants.

Bush and his team directed us away from some potential dangers and toward others, suggesting that our way of life, our "freedom," was under attack.

THE FEAR CAMPAIGN

Fear became a major theme of the 2004 presidential campaign. As Frank Rich wrote in the New York Times on July 25, 2004, "In the fear game, the Democrats are the visiting team, playing at a serious disadvantage. Out of power, they can't suit up officials at will to go on camera to scare us." They did the next best thing by nominating a war hero, playing this credential for all it was worth, while the Republicans seemed to be counting on the historically proven paradox that the less safe we felt, the more likely we would be to stick with a familiar face come Election Day. And even for those who claimed they wanted someone different, judging from Kerry's endorsement of the war on terror and Iraq, there was no indication that fearmongering would have been less prevalent in a Kerry administration.

"The leitmotif of the 2004 election is fear," John Harwood wrote in the Wall Street Journal on September 1, 2004. While Republicans were promoting Bush as the securer of safety and denigrating Kerry as "unfit for command," Democrats in turn were warning of the danger of another four years with Bush, especially with regard to civil liberties. The American Prospect, a leading reflector of liberal Democratic sentiment, was running covers depicting an elephant's trunk around the neck of the Statue of Liberty, and labeling Bush "the Most Dangerous President Ever."

The overall effect of this back-and-forth fearmongering was to make the public feel even more unsafe.

The perpetual promulgation of worst-case scenarios causes unnecessary panic. In the political context it is clear that this panic can be used both to control and to rally support. In Bush's famous speech to the nation on March 17, 2003, giving Hussein forty-eight hours to get out of town, Bush said, "The danger is clear: using chemical, biological, or, one day, nuclear weapons, obtained with the help of Iraq, the terrorists could . . . kill thousands or hundreds of thousands of innocent people in our country."

HOW THE GOVERNMENT BENEFITS FROM FEAR

A year later, in February 2004, days before Bush's Meet the Press interview with Tim Russert, Al Gore, casting himself as a non-alarmist among Democrats, gave the keynote speech at the three-day conference on fear at New School University. While Bush was getting ready to project his protector image to millions via Russert, Gore spoke to mere hundreds about how fear was used as rhetoric to help politicians like Bush stay in office.

Gore began by stating that the goal of terrorists was to cause a wave of fear out of proportion to the true danger. "Terrorism, after all, is the ultimate misuse of fear for political ends. Indeed, its specific goal is to distort the political reality of a nation by creating fear in the general population that is hugely disproportionate to the actual danger the terrorists are capable of posing."

Gore continued with an indictment of how Bush's rush to war was itself a form of terrorism. "President Bush and his administration have been force-feeding the American people a grossly exaggerated fear of Iraq that was hugely disproportionate to the actual danger posed by Iraq."

His former woodenness gone, Gore weighed his words carefully and hammered them out to the rapt audience that filled the auditorium or watched him from video screens in nearby rooms. He provided historical perspective, showing how fear of terrorists rather than from terrorists had been used throughout American history to justify restrictions of our liberties. Examples included the Alien and Sedition Acts of 1798, the internment of Japanese Americans in World War II, and the McCarthy abuses of the Cold War.

As former vice president Gore's talk drew to a conclusion, he provided a vision of hope that might free us from the sense of capitulation that fear politics demanded from us. He said, "There are only the politics of fear and the politics of trust. One says: 'You are encircled by monstrous dangers. Give us power over your freedom so we may protect you.' The other says: 'The world is a baffling and hazardous place, but it can be shaped to the will of men.'"

WHEN FEAR GRABS THE HEADLINES

The following morning, the fear conference reconvened in the same auditorium. This time there was a panel that included Joseph Ledoux, Barry

Glassner, a professor of sociology at the University of Southern California and the author of *The Culture of Fear*, and Tom Pyszczynski.

Barry Glassner was the speaker just before Dr. Pyszczynski, and whereas Pyszczynski described the essential importance of culture to house and sublimate our fears, Glassner went to extensive lengths to show that ours was a culture of deception, in which we were misdirected to the wrong dangers. If culture was crucial to reassure us, the culture of deception could make us more afraid.

Glassner, appearing youthful with a full head of black curls and thick black retro glasses, said that we live in the safest times in human history and that we are being manipulated by fear unnecessarily. Said Glassner, "Crime rates plunge, while surveys show Americans think crime rates are rising. At a time when people are living longer and healthier, people are worried about iffy illnesses." The media focus on particular aspects of a problem, inflating and distorting it until the audience has internalized the experience and considers the reported danger an accepted fact.

Glassner's book focused on the 1990s, and though his conclusions were applicable to the post-9/11 period, there had been an important change. American society felt more vulnerable, not so much because of 9/11 itself as because of the extensive media coverage of it. The mushrooming of cable news coverage since 9/11 had added an important amplifier to the problem.

Amplification had been used repeatedly to hype potential contagions in the post-9/11 world, beginning with anthrax, in which the free-floating anxiety of 9/11 was transferred to a hysterical fear of our mail.

The fear apparatus was less pervasive before 9/11, though it was growing in that period. Said Glassner, "Between 1990 and 1998, the murder rate decreased by 20 percent, while murder stories on media newscasts increased by 600 percent (not even counting O. J. Simpson). Isolated incidents are treated as trends. Fearmongering focused on youth violence. In the 1980s and '90s, politicians and journalists acted as if just about every young American was a potential mass murderer, despite the actual decrease in murders. In 1996 and '97, fear was tied to school violence—William Bennett called it the violence of 'super predators.' Yet urban crime continued to drop, so the media was finally compelled to change its jargon to talk about isolated murders in suburban and rural areas. But three times more kids were killed by lightning than violence. The Columbine murders were unprecedented, but for twelve months before there was nothing. Less than 1 percent of homicides occur in or around schools."

Bureaucrats used fear by playing Chicken Little. They could claim at every turn that a disaster might be coming, thereby keeping their budgets high and avoiding blame should disaster really strike.

OUR PROTECTOR

On December 21, 2003, four days before Christmas, Tom Ridge, who served as homeland security secretary during Bush's first term, had raised the terror alert status back to orange, which meant a high risk of a terrorist attack over the remainder of the holiday season in the United States. There were several reasons given for this announcement: the increased buzz and threats circulating among al-Qaeda members, the fact that this terrorist group tended to strike on an every-other-year basis, plus the logic that we were more vulnerable as a country with increased travel taking place during the holiday season.

Along with this announcement came the headline that it was intended not to spread fear but to encourage preparation. Somehow we would be sending a message back to al-Qaeda that we were ready for them.

But no one out on the streets really knew how to conceptualize this. Was al-Qaeda coming? When and where? The alert had been raised many times, but many of us didn't know how to respond. We had gotten used to the warnings, but the possibility of an attack could still caused some nervousness.

Since 9/11, many of us had become more apprehensive overall. Like Dr. Sabban's rats, once alerted, we were more easily frightened a second time, or a third. Of course, worrywarts in places like Idaho and Montana didn't have New York and Washington's sense of vulnerability to begin with, no matter how much cable news they watched.

Many in the United States had a false sense of security before 9/11. With the exception of the War of 1812, our continent had never been invaded while the American flag flew over it. The 9/11 attacks happened suddenly and opened us up to feelings of vulnerability that countries like Russia and Israel were more accustomed to. Over time, even if we gained a better perspective and learned to redefine our personal risk as low, still, the worldwide interconnection of our media outlets via satellite and Internet practically assured that the bug du jour, or the scare of the moment, would instantly escalate into worldwide concern via the media megaphone.

The sense of fear in the United States in the early part of the 21st century seemed as high or higher than at the height of the Cold War, when the Soviet Union had its enormous arsenal of nuclear weapons aimed at us.

Why? The greatest reason for the change was the growing fracturing and parceling of information into hyped media sound bites. No matter how safe we were, all we needed to hear was the word danger or threat, and the cycle of worry started. When one cycle was extinguished, another one took its place.

In the post-9/11 world, the only cable station that didn't scare us was the cartoon channel, which lacked headlines or news updates of any kind. However, in January 2004, I even noted on the cartoon channel a shift in the wrong direction, when "Grandpa" on Hey, Arnold! told the other characters that they'd better "watch out for weapons of mass destruction."

SAFETY SPEAK

The New York Police Department sent a memo to the staff at my medical center on December 23, 2003. It was filled with the kinds of warnings quickly becoming ubiquitous in New York City. It was the new safety speak. It included sage advice on how to be on the lookout for a terrorist. The criteria for a suspected terrorist included someone who wore baggy clothing or who exhibited nervousness or extreme concentration, tunnel vision or singular determination, and perspiration. At NYU Medical Center, this description might fit a typical medical student.

NEW YEAR'S EVE 2004

With the holiday season approaching, terrorism fears were once again hyped. Homeland Security Secretary Ridge announced that he had good information that an attack was imminent, and we were back on orange alert nationwide. Here in New York City, we had never left orange, and we had long been used to seeing police with sniffing dogs and even National Guardsmen in combat fatigues at the entrances to our tunnels and bridges.

On Christmas Day 2003, Eric Lichtblau and Craig Smith of the New York Times reported that officials were tightening airport security from Paris to Los Angeles. CNN advised its viewers to go about their usual holiday plans while at the same time reporting that terrorists might once again attack a prominent U.S. target by hijacking an airplane.

In France, Air France canceled six flights between Paris and Los Angeles at the urging of United States officials, who said they suspected that up to a half-dozen passengers on the flights had "links to terrorism." In Chicago, officials imposed flight restrictions over downtown at the request of the mayor's office, blocking small aircraft below three thousand feet for fear the Sears Tower might be hit. Officials at Los Angeles International Airport banned passengers from being picked up or dropped off at the terminal curb. The intelligence agencies were reportedly most concerned about flights originating in France and Mexico based on terrorism intelligence, or chatter, gleaned from electronic spying as well as informants.

Jet fighters patrolled our skies and others were on alert, but rather than make us feel safer, it caused many of us to worry.

On December 31, Flight 490 from Mexico to the United States was canceled because American officials felt it might be the target of an attack, and then on New Year's Day, British Airways Flight 223, which was scheduled to embark for Dulles Airport in Washington, D.C., was canceled after British government officials warned the airline of security concerns, according to the New York Times. This same flight had been the subject of concern a day earlier, when it was accompanied to Dulles by F-16s, and the passengers were questioned upon landing. Again on Friday, January 2, 2004, Flight 223 was canceled and kept on the ground in London.

On New Year's Eve, I was in Fort Lauderdale with my family. We were supposed to depart for New York's LaGuardia airport at 8:30 P.M., but the plane was held in Boston for "security reasons." We were assigned another plane but had to wait for the pilots to arrive from Boston to fly us to New York. The Boston plane finally arrived at 11:15 P.M., but even after we boarded the new plane, it was held until after midnight before departing. We were told that we were still waiting for the pilots, though I had seen them come off the Boston plane. It was clear to me—as well as to several other passengers—that we were being held on the ground until after midnight while New York was being watched.

This type of precaution, without being told the reasons behind it or the information that the government was acting on, caused a hum of nervousness to pervade airports everywhere on New Year's Eve. Unease and uncertainty caused us to be afraid.

Our government wanted its citizens to know that it was protecting us. But the way the information was being parceled out followed by the jarring media announcements made us worry automatically.

No matter what the reason for the alerts, they made us worry far more than we needed to in order to protect ourselves. We could ignore them, but we could never stop worrying entirely once the first fight-or-flight response had been triggered.

PREPARATIONS

In early 2004, I discussed our readiness for terrorism with my neighbor Dr. Leon Pachter, back then the head of the trauma service at New York University and Bellevue. He had stood outside Bellevue with me on September 11, 2001, waiting for the potential survivors who never came, and he had since volunteered his time to help organize an emergency response system in New York City.

"Forget it," he said. "Since September 11, there's been no real preparation. Doctors and so-called first responders are no more organized now than they were back then."

I shook my head. First the government and the media exaggerate a potential threat; then they try to show that they are protecting us from it; then we discover that the protection is faulty, and we become even more afraid.

It was a good thing that Dr. Pachter's comments weren't publicized. If the news media got hold of quotes like his, it might cause yet another unnecessary panic.

Instead, the New York Times headlined the opposite news on February 15, 2004, claiming that "New York Police Take Broad Steps in Facing Terror." I was more inclined to believe Pachter, especially since the Times was using mostly unnamed sources. This article attempted to show how extensive preparations were being made by the police in conjunction with "city health officials" and "federal authorities."

Training reportedly involved potential plans to board cruise ships, and there was a plan in the works to test the city's air for biological agents, and to provide antibiotics and vaccines if necessary. Another drill prepared the coroner's office for dealing with corpses contaminated from chemical weapons.

New sophisticated detection devices included a system that would detect the presence of more than a hundred different viruses or bacteria within forty-five minutes. Since poor New York didn't yet have this latest technology, it was forced to rely in the meantime on Biowatch, a system whereby ten "nondescript monitors" would "sniff the air for fifteen lethal pathogens," with an alarming twenty-four-hour delay for processing results. Oldstyle radiation detectors were reportedly being used throughout the city. Two hundred distribution centers were also being planned so that as many as eight million people could receive emergency treatment in five to ten days' time, relying on the federal stockpile of vaccines and drugs. If a quarantine should prove necessary, city health officials were ready "to persuade New Yorkers exposed to a deadly infectious pathogen to stay at home."

But this lavish outdated display—even if it actually existed—was likely to be of little use. These science-fictionesque measures were designed for an almost inconceivable worst-case scenario. Instead of feeling protected, people I knew who read the Times article immediately broke into a cold sweat.

OLD AND RECURRENT THREATS

On Monday, August 2, 2004, a terror alert was issued that financial centers in some of our major cities, including New York, were under direct threat by al-Qaeda. Police presence increased visibly, traffic thickened, and people everywhere wondered whether they were about to be attacked. President Bush predictably announced, "We are a country in danger. We are doing everything we can to confront this danger."

The alert was based on the computer files and related information uncovered following the arrest of an al-Qaeda operative in Pakistan.

By Tuesday it was determined that much of the information released was in fact three or four years old, and there was no evidence that a terror plot was actually underway.

The New York Times, the Washington Post, and other major newspapers, after splattering the initial concerns over their front pages on Monday, on Tuesday sheepishly front-paged the qualifying information. And a Tuesday Times editorial read, "But it's unfortunate that it is necessary to fight suspicions of political timing, suspicions the administration has sown by misleading the public on security."

Once again the public appeared to have been thrown into a fight-or-flight mode unnecessarily. Once again, unlike animals, we were transmitting danger signals based on abstract information. Abstract risk assessment is an advantage for humans over animals only as long as we can learn to use it accurately.

Agenda-driven communication creates a problem with a basic mechanism such as fear. The al-Qaeda report was overpersonalized, the danger perceived was out of proportion to the real risk, and the fear response was useless or even maladaptive.

By Wednesday, government officials, including Tom Ridge, the secretary of homeland security at the time, tried to salvage the situation by saying that al-Qaeda took a long time to size up and stalk a potential target. But by this time, the public imagination was already diverted, though the fear of al-Qaeda remained just below the surface.

In fact, in a final pre-election ad, the Bush campaign cast the terrorist threat as menacing wolves prowling through a shadowy forest. They knew well by this point that our attention might have on-and-off switch, but our fear did not.

5

FALSE EVIDENCE, ASSUMED RISK

We are hard-wired in our brains to fear first, think second.

—David Ropeik

FALSE EVIDENCE

Joey Reynolds, the host of a late-night talk show for many years on WOR radio in New York, anointed fear "False Evidence Assumed Risk." "Fear," he said to me, "occurs when you don't think you can get what you need." Reynolds said many people deal with their own fear of personal loss by making others afraid in their place. "And no matter how inaccurate, the greater the impact, the more powerful the scarer feels."

Reynolds was radio's version of the counter person at the deli, and for many years he lulled thousands of anxious insomniacs to sleep every night with his peculiar lullabies. His guests were like guests in his living room, and he served them food and coffee as any generous host would.

I asked Reynolds if he thought we could become used to this fear over time, become desensitized to it, and evolve into better-balanced human beings despite our fragmented media-driven lives. He laughed his knowing cackle and said he didn't see how we could.

SPINNING FEAR

Narratives were employed by the mainstream media to advance a story, embodying aspects of fiction in order to hold their audiences' attention.

These narratives tend to be compatible with others already in circulation. According to Barry Glassner, prior to 2001, a "sick society" narrative predominated. In this story, heroes were hard to find, and villains were domestic. The story line was ultimately about the decline of Western civilization.

Post-9/11, there was a new narrative. In this story, people were pulling together to fight a common enemy, villains were from foreign lands, and Americans were the object of scorn of the rest of the world. In this narrative, former villains were now portrayed as heroes, including the previously criticized fire department and police.

After a few years, the media was growing weary of the new narrative. The country was dividing into factions, no longer pulling together, and our leaders were once again perceived by many as villains worth discrediting, and Western civilization was once again seen as declining.

Despite this shift in emphasis, one strategy remained the same throughout all the narratives: newspapers, television, and radio continued to exaggerate minor dangers.

The risk terrain had changed. Trustworthy mentors who put things in perspective for us had been largely replaced by the bright lights of computer and TV screens that offered info fragments, alarming us more often than they reassured. This was the new topography of worry. Go-to people had almost disappeared. We had lost the ability to assess risk. Our ability to judge real danger was impaired.

THE PROPER USE OF FEAR

In 1997, Gavin de Becker published *The Gift of Fear*, a book about how to use fear properly. He described fears that protect. Perhaps most important, he warned against the destructive power of prolonged states of unremitting fear. "Far too many people are walking around in a constant state of vigilance, their intuition misinformed about what really poses danger. It needn't be so. . . . Real fear is a signal intended to be very brief, a mere servant of intuition."

Some of de Becker's examples were extreme. The experience of being stalked by a murderer, or of being famous and the vulnerable object of adoring fans, was not something that most of us could, or should try to, relate to. But many people have tried to break off a relationship only to have the jilted suitor stalk them. "There's a lesson in real-life stalking cases. The fact that a romantic pursuer is relentless doesn't mean you are special— it means he (or she) is troubled." This kind of fear radar is not hype but protective. If someone in an intimate relationship feels intuitively that he or she is at risk, it is often the case, especially if the partner has a history of violence. De Becker pointed out that a partner's "justifications for violence" and threats are always to be taken seriously.

De Becker wrote convincingly that recognizing real danger is the key to real safety. He told the story of a woman who had just been raped who somehow sensed that she was about to be killed. De Becker called it a survival signal—when the perpetrator closed the window just when he said he was about to leave, the victim's unconscious signaled her into a fight-or-flight mode, and she sneaked away just as he went into her kitchen to find a knife. The closed window was a sign that the perpetrator didn't want the noise of the murder to be overheard. Previous to this she had been submissive, controlled by the violence, but with the closing of the window, her unconscious was alerted. With no time left, she rallied to take back control and escape.

De Becker was an expert in telling the difference between "a real warning and mere words." "If your intuition is informed accurately, the danger signal will sound when it should. If you come to trust this fact, you'll not only be safer, but it will be possible to live life nearly free of fear."

In 2002, in the post-9/11 climate, de Becker wrote a follow-up book: Fear Less. He concluded that despite the terrorist attacks we could still feel safe, in part by understanding our enemies were not "superhuman," but "merely anti-human." "Occasionally effective, to be sure, but our enemies are not powerful or ubiquitous."

"Many of us tend to think of the world in terms of good guys and bad guys. Bad guys help create our fears. Good guys help us feel protected. Unfortunately, our concern about bad guys is often blown out of proportion to the real danger they represent."

"After 9/11, we went through an adjustment period. We recognized that violence could happen to us. Many of us began to imagine worst-case scenarios involving weapons and terrorists, or we were handed them by the media. Wrote de Becker, "But if a person feels fear constantly, there is no signal left for when it's really needed. Thus, the person who chooses to worry all the time or to persistently chew on unwarranted fears is actually making himself less safe . . . trusting intuition is the exact opposite of living in fear. When you honor intuitive signals and evaluate them without denial, you can actually relax, even in these troubled times."

Post-9/11, the group of people who were covered by the debris of the falling World Trade Center expanded to include practically the entire country, as we were all bombarded by media images of destruction and fear of further terrorism. This fear was contagious. Many of us vacillated between feelings of disbelief and panic. Hyped symptoms of posttraumatic stress that included helplessness, numbness, and withdrawal from daily activities lasted for weeks.

The TV generation that grew up in America watching Wile E. Coyote zoom unhindered off countless cartoon cliffs in Roadrunner episodes, and later became watchers of building-crushing flicks such as The Towering Inferno and Independence Day, experienced an initial detachment from the real events of September 11, 2001. To many baby boomers, the balls of fire and the thunderous crash didn't seem real. But as the news media continued their focus, the horror began to sink in, which helped fuel an outpouring of concern and generosity as people everywhere banded together. Yet the news coverage also caused countless people who had lost no one to feel vulnerable and afraid. This wasn't true posttraumatic stress, since most of us hadn't experienced the trauma directly, but many personalized it and felt helpless. It was only over time, by sticking to family, to work, to passions, that we began to live normal lives again.

Dr. Rachel Yehuda, an expert on posttraumatic stress, told me she thinks we struggled as a society in this period because we felt entitled to live a trauma-free life. We said, "Why me?" whereas "in a previous generation, no one had the expectation that something wouldn't happen to them—in those days, it was 'Why not me?' Previously, no one thought that being exposed to a trauma was that unusual."

"Posttraumatic stress is a mismatch between what we think the world should be like, and what it is really like. We aren't prepared. In a culture where you're expecting people to hate you, you let go of it for a lot longer. In Europe, for example, Jews always had the thought that a certain percentage wouldn't survive because of anti-Semitism. There was a lower expectation of peaceful existence, so the trauma of threat was less."

Dr. Yehuda also indicated that many of our scientists and those who inform us do us a disservice by overdramatizing their concerns. This grandiosity is part of what causes the public to over perceive risks. "We scientists can't tolerate being cogs in a wheel. Technology allows us to look at things we never could before. But we need to learn to be excited by what we do without telling a premature story. We can alarm people unnecessarily. And then we're stuck with our story, right or wrong."

ASSESSING RISK

We needed to learn how to see risk in perspective, without overreacting to imagined dangers. Unfortunately, there was no consensus about what constituted proper risk assessment or the best way to accomplish it. There was disagreement about who is an expert on risk, and some authors don't trust so-called experts at all because of their hidden agendas.

Published in 2002, David Ropeik and George Gray's book Risk was a practical guide intended to counter the hysteria caused by inaccurate public health reporting. Like de Becker, these authors believed that "we live in a dangerous world. Yet it was also a world far safer in many ways than it has ever been. Life expectancy is up. Infant mortality is down. Diseases that only recently were mass killers have been all but eradicated. Advances in public health, medicine, environmental regulation, food safety, and worker protection have dramatically reduced many of the major risks we faced just a few decades ago."

Ropeik and Gray developed a risk meter, a way of converting uncertainty into calculable risk. This risk meter assesses the likelihood of exposure to a potential danger as well as the consequences if you are one of the unlucky victims. The list of risks is extensive. Accidents, alcohol, tobacco, and obesity top the list in terms of both prevalence and severity of outcome. On the other end of the spectrum, vaccines are deemed essentially safe, mad cow disease is too rare in humans to be a factor, mercury doesn't really affect most people, and pesticides have a minimal impact.

The book attempted to reorient the reader. The authors would see dangers demystified. Their goal was to cut the public loose from hype and decontaminate us from prior misconceptions.

But Cass Sunstein, founder and director of the Program on Behavioral Economics and Public Policy at Harvard Law School, distrusted authorities who approached us with a "we know what's best for you" attitude. In 2002, Sunstein published the book Risk and Reason, in which he suggested that it is not the expert or official, but the populist/consumer advocate who generally has our best interests at heart. Sunstein would likely distrust Ropeik and Gray's fear meters as simplistic and too easily politicized, preferring instead the judgment of the same consumer advocates that Ropeik and Gray might see as inaccurate. According to Sunstein, "Populists insist that the very characterization of risks involves no simple 'fact,' . . . In the populist view . . . any judgment about risk is subjective . . . for populists, ordinary intuitions have normative force."

Like Ropeik and Gray, Sunstein also observed that information about risk was easily distorted, but unlike the authors of Risk, Sunstein generally blamed the government. He wrote, "Public officials know that they might be severely punished for downplaying a risk that is perceived as serious or for calling attention to a hazard that is perceived as trivial . . . to avoid charges of insensitivity . . . he [the public official] may make speeches and promote policies that convey deep concern about the very waste spill that he actually considers harmless." The effective politician rides the waves from one created danger to the next: "Thus people might be fearful, for a time, about some risk—shark attacks, or air travel in the aftermath of a disaster—that produces no concern at all after a few months."

As Bruce Schneier, a world-respected security expert, wrote in his 2003 book Beyond Fear, "When you're living in fear, it's easy to let others make decisions for you. . . . To get beyond fear, you have to start thinking intelligently about the trade-offs you make. You have to start evaluating the risks you face." Taking responsibility for our own fear meter sometimes means disregarding public pronouncements of risks, while at other times accepting them.

But Schneier was also concerned that we could too easily give up our freedom to a blanket authority that promised to handle our risk assessment for us but ultimately didn't make us more secure, in part because this authority tended to magnify threats. Like Sunstein, Schneier did not trust the usual experts and officials to advise us or protect us.

Wrote Schneier, "We are told that we are in graver danger than ever, and that we must change our lives in drastic and inconvenient ways in order to be secure. We are told that we must sacrifice privacy and anonymity and accept restrictions on our actions. We are told that the police need new far-reaching investigative powers, that domestic spying capabilities need to be instituted, and that we must spy on each other. . . . But the reality is that most of the changes we're being asked to endure won't result in good security. . . . Even in the worst neighborhoods, most people are safe. It's hard to find a terrorist, kidnapper, bank robber, because there simply aren't that many in our society."

So we can't trust our risk experts no matter who they are because their views depend on their agendas. But this doesn't mean we can automatically trust our intuition either, which, as de Becker wrote, is too often "misinformed." Any resolution of this dichotomy between misinforming experts and misguided intuition must involve retraining in how to recognize danger.

FINDING THINGS TO FEAR

On September 24, 2003, Anne Applebaum addressed the American terrain of worry in a column titled "Finding Things to Fear" in the Washington Post. She too was arguing against the wisdom of our unschooled intuition.

She described how we have miscalculated risks in the post-9/11 world because of our continuing anxiety. "After Sept. 11, 2001, thousands of people in this country swore off airplanes and began driving cars, apparently believing that cars are safer. In fact, the number of deaths on U.S. highways in a typical year—more than 40,000—is more than double the number of people who have died in all commercial airplane accidents in the past 40 years. To put it differently, the odds of being killed in a terrorist incident in 2002 were 1 in 9 million. In that same year, the odds of dying in a traffic accident were about 1 in 7,000. By taking the precaution of not flying, many people died."

Indeed, we were far safer in America, but we felt more afraid. We Americans had dramatically reduced our risk in every area of life, and our life spans were 60 percent longer in 2000 than in 1900. We had thousands of safety devices, including smoke detectors, circuit breakers, and air bags. We were protected against everyday mishaps of all kinds. Yet if our fears weren't real, we invented them.

THE GOOD GUYS

Without mentors, without people we could trust, we grew more fearful. Doctors were among the groups of former good guys who had been discredited by our culture of worry. At the outset of the twenty-first century, patients were frightened by the latest technologies, but even more so by the impersonal and robotic way medical information was sometimes delivered. In the context of today's fear-provoking parceling out of health factoids, a well-informed communicative caring physician—a throwback to an earlier time in history—could make a big difference in calming fears and providing perspective.

The television character Marcus Welby was a paradigm of the kind of physician I'm referring to, who above all else offered a dose of reassurance and perspective to the dispensing of treatment. It is no accident that the Welby TV show reruns faded from the screen over the years, and even with the propagation of cable stations, this old medical show is still rarely seen. It is no wonder that ratings-obsessed TV got rid of Welby for being out-of-date, realizing that today's time-constrained doctors have too little in common with the hand-holders of yesteryear.

Marcus Welby, M.D., at the time a very popular medical drama set in middle America, ran from 1969 to 1976 on ABC. Robert Young as Welby was a study in bedside manner. The creased brow of concern, the empathetic pat on the patient's shoulder, these Welby trademarks delivered the message that a family doctor could guide a patient caringly through life's crises. Marcus Welby, M.D. was a response to the beginning of the technological age. In an era that celebrated the invention of coronary bypass surgery, a revolutionary procedure that didn't require hand-holding, Welby believed in comforting the patient as much as curing the illness.

In a movie that emphasized Welby's obsolescence, The Return of Marcus Welby, in 1984, a hospital tried to cut the privileges of its oldest doctors, including Welby. He argued ineffectively that a patient would be lost among the CT scanners, the MRIs, and the multitude of pills.

In the worried post-9/11 world, there was a surge of volunteerism among physicians that brought back memories of the old Welby house-call days. Unfortunately, this return to an era of physician guidance was short-lived, and we all soon went back to rushing for clipped fees from one worried patient to the next.

But in smiling old Doc Welby's world, there was no withholding of information or ignoring the frightened patient. The doctor battled a puzzling illness until the diagnosis was made, and the patient was attended to until he or she felt comfortable.

THE BAD GUYS

Though we were often afraid of people who didn't directly threaten us, at the same time, in the rare instance when we encountered someone who was truly dangerous, we might not know how to identify him. With all the unnecessary worry we experience, there was still no guarantee that the real bad guys wouldn't slip by us. In fact, perhaps if we weren't casting such a wide safety net, we might be more likely to notice a clear danger signal, like a pilot in training who said he didn't need to know how to land.

The good Arthur R. Droba, J.D., M.D., was an internist who performed insurance screening physicals for the FAA in Sarasota, Florida. He examined the 9/11 terrorist leader Mohammed Atta and okayed him to fly. Afterward, he couldn't remember his infamous patient, though his nurse had heard him say he felt Atta was a "bad man."

Droba's friend Arne Kruithof was the forty-year-old director of the flight school in Sarasota that trained Ziyad Al-Jarrah, one of the hijackers of Flight 93. Kruithof found this Machiavellian pilot-to-be honest, hardworking, well mannered, and intelligent.

Al-Jarrah's own father, the minister of social affairs in Lebanon, and his uncle, the director of a large bank, said they couldn't believe he had done such a thing.

Terrorists were hard to recognize. They didn't wear the mark of Cain on their foreheads.

Kruithof said to me in an interview that he felt horrible about not seeing Al-Jarrah's evil. "German intelligence had tracked him in Hamburg, meeting with Atta. He was in Afghanistan for a few weeks. He wasn't there on a charity mission."

I suggested that there was also a Dostoyevskian phenomenon to consider, the over-intellectualization of political acts. In Crime and Punishment, the protagonist Raskolnikov kills an aged woman to test his theory that someone who makes others' lives miserable doesn't deserve to live.

Kruithof considered the comparison between Raskolnikov and his fledgling pilot. "When I looked into his eyes," he said finally, "I saw someone intelligent, perhaps too intelligent for our society. Someone who is bitter and cold. Someone who passes by an old man who can't walk anymore and decides the man should be subtracted from the equation for walking so slow. The cause was more important than the life."

I asked Kruithof if there was some way to pick out a terrorist, someone who intends you great harm. He paused, considering my question. In America we saw terrorists everywhere we looked, but he had known a real one.

"Al-Jarrah dressed well," he said. "He looked European. Good social manners. He was hard to spot. He was slow at times, but he trained up to a commercial level."

Kruithof sighed heavily. "You think it's someone you like, who you used to hang out with. It's hard for the brain to accept what happened."

Kruithof witnessed up close the danger that we just imagined. He, like the rest of us, lacked an accurate fear radar.

SARS:
THE FIRST CORONAVIRUS
OUTBREAK

It seemed . . . very easy to paint the worst-case scenario.
I thought about this, how our minds naturally jump
to picture the negative outcome and stall there. It is because
the mind is frozen by fear, and fear overwhelms hope.

—Jerome Groopman, M.D., *The Anatomy of Hope*

In April 2003 up rose SARS to grab the media megaphone. SARS, or Severe Acute Respiratory Syndrome, brought the panic over a potential infection to a new level. The global health alert and travel advisories that were meant to inhibit the dissemination of the virus also spread virulent fear by word of mouth. Public health agencies raised the stakes, then presumptively took credit for the resolution of the problem.

The government sounded its note of preparedness, wanting to seem proactive in another public panic situation where it was actually being reactive. The CDC, which had lost credibility with the anthrax bungle in 2001, rallied publicly with SARS and public health quarantined entire sections of the planet in response to a virus that demonstrated seven thousand cases worldwide. The CDC and the World Health Organization (WHO) used fear to provoke compliance, talking about worst-case scenarios and viral mutations, and alarming the whole Western Hemisphere beginning with a few cases that flew around a Toronto hotel.

But no one died of SARS in the United States in 2003, though close to 800 did die worldwide. The CDC and the World Health Organization restricted travel to and from Asia and Toronto based on the correct assumption that air travel could allow an emerging contagion especially a respiratory virus to spread more easily. Historically, isolating an afflicted patient had always been the first step and regional quarantines for plague, influenza, other contagious threats throughout history had been effective but carried significant costs. People tended to panic from an imposed quarantine which could help spread a bug. It was human nature to run away from perceived risk and human nature to make common mistakes when engaged in hypervigilant activity. People who faced heavy stigmatizing for being a suspected disease carrier could lose their common sense altogether.

When the incidence of SARS died down (as many emerging viruses had done before it), the health organizations were quick to give the credit to their worldwide advisory.

THE CHOKEHOLD

Back in early April 2003, President Bush granted Secretary of Health and Human Services Tommy Thompson the right to quarantine for SARS.

In its more than fifty years of existence, the WHO had never before issued a travel advisory or enacted a global surveillance network, as it did with SARS. In the United States, meanwhile, the CDC was publicly analyzing every conceivable case—another unprecedented reaction. SARS was a legitimate concern, though by April, the virus had infected about two thousand people worldwide and killed fewer than one hundred, compared to the yearly average influenza death toll of thirty-six thousand in the United States alone.

What was going on medically? The answer was complex, since the SARS corona virus was a cousin to the common cold, which spread easily via sneezing or even touch. But SARS was much more severe, causing inflammation in the lungs. And we had no immunity to it.

A strong public health initiative seemed warranted. As Julie Gerberding, then the director of the CDC, pointed out in the New England Journal of Medicine, the cooperation of the international scientific community in identifying the corona virus as the culprit in a matter of weeks was very impressive. But Gerberding didn't stop with the scientists. She wrote: "Even more impressive than the speed of scientific discovery in the global SARS outbreak is the almost instantaneous communication and information exchange that has supported every aspect of the response."

She was right, though the result of all the communication was global panic in addition to containment and economic shutdown that carried enormous costs.

The WHO was heavily involved. In fact the Chinese government suppressed information initially, but the international health community, with the WHO involved and with boots on the ground in the Spring of 2003, helped to pressure the Chinese medical authorities to take their heads out of the sand, identify patients, and isolate true cases.

The travel restrictions on top of this clearly helped to slow the spread of the virus. Gerberding as the new director of the CDC was giving speeches and press conferences. SARS was a full-fledged international bug du jour, with news and media coverage beyond any predecessor. The WHO was involved with global tracking strategies utilizing improved technology, greater scientific cooperation, and an increased interest in tracking infectious agents because of concern over possible bioterrorism.

But there was soon a down side where the public began to perceive too much emphasis on public statements and not as much on serological testing and antiviral strategies. SARS needed to be cured with laboratory work, not press conferences. Panic over SARS grew along with focus on the worst case scenario.

This helped to spread worldwide economic havoc—many estimates were that SARS cost over $30 billion to local economies worldwide. Toronto was cut off by the WHO travel advisory throughout much of April 2003.

Chinatowns were deserted in all the major cities, and people around the world were stigmatizing anyone who came from an Asian country. Xenophobia grew.

In contrast to the rest of Asia, Vietnam's careful and quiet isolating of suspected patients seemed to be behind its success in limiting the spread of the virus. Quarantining hospitals where SARS had spread to health care workers, or designating certain centers as "SARS hospitals," was at the upper limit of what seemed reasonable. Monitoring of traffic from countries where SARS had been diagnosed, or emphasizing careful precautions in such countries, was also reasonable but was not the same thing as frightening everyone who may have traveled there.

The problem with AIDS information back in the 1980s had been the opposite kind of distortion: affected groups were marginalized, and the prevailing rhetoric had downplayed the disease. With SARS, the propaganda was fear, suggesting that everyone could get it overnight, which was far from the case. This notion had a negative impact on many people. Physician/essayist Abraham Verghese, writing in the New York Times Magazine, attacked the transparent political agendas that had been applied to bioterror preparation but made an invalid assumption that none of this applied to SARS. Certainly, restricting movement was necessary with a known killer, but with SARS, people were restricted throughout the spring of 2003 just for having a cough. Many life insurance companies wouldn't grant a person a policy if he'd been anywhere near Asia in the past month. This was an overreaction.

The distinction had to be made between the need for global control of a virus before it got out of hand and the political agenda of people wanting to justify their jobs and project themselves as soothsayers. The machinery for public broadcasting that had been set up for bioterror prevention was being used indiscriminately for SARS. It was a blind assumption that speaking about SARS incessantly on TV would prevent its spread.

GALVANIZING FEAR

The greatest problem with SARS was public health authorities speaking too much about worst-case scenarios as a justification for large expenditures. Attention paid to SARS took attention and resources away from AIDS, malaria, influenza, and tuberculosis. Fear came from not knowing exactly where SARS came from, though its bat origin and a civet cat was eventually established, the knowledge helping to calm fears.

Still, we had no immunity to SARS, and we had no vaccine.

The lead question in doctor's offices throughout April 2003 was what people should do to protect themselves against SARS. The answer of course was to do absolutely nothing. The best vaccine for SARS was information, seeing the new disease in its context. At the time there were only thirty-five documented cases in the United States, and no one had died. We had to treat the perception that we could get SARS rather than any real risk of it. We needed to convert our uncertainty to a realistic understanding of our chances of getting the disease, which were extremely low for any given individual.

How did a person know if he had SARS? The answer was that if he had a fever, muscle aches, and difficulty breathing, he didn't have SARS, but he probably had the flu.

A FEAR OF ASIANS

The small waiting room in my office three blocks from my hospital was just as congested as the rest of New York, with patients sitting practically on top of one another. As with the subway, it felt as if germs here might spread more quickly than at other places, and I always half-expected my patients to catch the bug their neighbor was harboring. But whether the risk of catching something from another patient was real or imagined, one thing was certain: the stress of living and working in the city made it seem so. Added to this mix, in the spring of 2003 we had the seemingly tangible risk of SARS. My waiting room was filled with patients, all brimming with the same question.

"Could I have SARS?" a patient blurted out. Unsolicited, an office secretary replied, "You must ask the doctor." Meanwhile, the thirteen-inch television set in the middle of the room was playing all SARS all the time and updating my patients on the virus every hour.

An Asian American architect, "Mr. Ho," had come to see me for the first time. No one sat next to him in the waiting room, and when he coughed, the room emptied out altogether.

In my examination room, Mr. Ho announced that he had just returned from Hong Kong. He traveled to China and Hong Kong on business every few weeks, but because of the effect of the SARS scare on the economy there, he had lost his latest architectural job and had had to come back. On the plane bringing him home, he said, no one would sit with him.

He came to me with a cough and symptoms of a cold, but no fever, no muscle aches, no difficulty breathing. Hearing this, I wanted to don a mask, but I put on gloves instead. My patient downplayed his symptoms, clearly realizing I—the doctor—might be worried about SARS.

"It's just a cold," he said. "It was going away, then it came back a little. It's only a tickle."

Without saying the magic word, I reassured him that what he had sounded not like something sinister but like simple bronchitis. I gave him an antibiotic and sent him home.

Afterwards, I was suddenly nervous, thinking of my two young children. Doctors are not immune to worries about contagion. In my case the concern didn't go away completely until I had taken a shower and irrationally washed away the psychological remnant of my fear. It was the same thing I used to do for AIDS in the 1980s, scrubbing my hands after every encounter with every potential AIDS patient.

A week later, Ho returned to the office with a smile rather than a cough. During that week, the specter of SARS had spread through the world more rapidly than even the disease itself. Though not a single new case had been reported in our city, New Yorkers were increasingly frightened and increasingly wary.

Asia was more isolated than before, and Ho had no immediate prospect for work there. Back in New York, he thought people were taking into account his Asian features and avoiding him on the street. I could actually see this occurring in my waiting room, where the other patients now deliberately avoided not only him but anything he touched. This was awful and inexcusable.

So why was Ho smiling? In my consultation room he confessed that he had actually been afraid he had SARS, but now that he knew he didn't, despite the fact that he was not working, he believed his future was bright.

SARS IN NEW YORK CITY

New Yorkers are a nervous bunch to begin with, and our doctors are no exception. Most of us, doctors and patients alike, are medical Zeligs; like Woody Allen's character, we take on the symptoms and even the personality of the latest threat. The stress of living in an overcrowded city distorts perceptions in the direction of fear.

The scientific literature analyzing the health of our city's residents shows that a disproportionately high percentage of New York teenagers suffer from eating disorders related to a higher level of stress. The same literature shows that proportionately more adults suffer from heart disease for the same reason. After studying this phenomenon, the journal Psychosomatic Medicine reported in 1999 that these conditions are due to the strain of life in New York itself.

New Yorkers try to compensate for the pressure we feel by paying more attention to our symptoms, to every itch and twinge, as if this vigilance might protect us from an ever hostile environment. Our fear management is neurotic. Forever on the verge of panic, we seek out doctors more often and try to use elaborate health care safety nets to protect us from the ultimate free fall. The Journal of Urban Health in December 2002 described how New York's megacity has built an elaborate health system.

Our megacity also has more media than anywhere else, and so we are more quickly saturated and prodded by the latest hype. We feel the strain earlier but then we use our extensive safety net to become desensitized more quickly to the latest bug du jour, only to find ourselves right on the front lines of the next scare. It's a real roller-coaster ride.

In the era of SARS fear, we eventually developed a new sort of schtick. Though New Yorkers always cough and kvetch, I'd never heard so much nervous coughing before. We always seem to be on the verge of catching something, or if not actually catching something, at least complaining that we might. In the spring of 2003, each raspy breath seemed more significant, each sniffling acquaintance seemed ominously afflicted.

My office phone rang continually with respiratory complaints. I knew better than to counter these concerns with the bald statistic of zero deaths from SARS in the United States. I didn't want to appear to be downplaying serious potential risk even if that risk was remote at the time.

After a month of SARS worry, New Yorkers began building up an immunity to the fear.

According to the Centers for Disease Control, there were only two probable cases of SARS in New York City by May of 2003, cases that ultimately turned out not to be SARS. So our respiratory filters joined our gas masks and our stash of antibiotics in our tiny closets.

Unfortunately, we would come to need our masks many years later.

SARS WHEN THE SMOKE CLEARED

By July of 2003, long after it had dropped off the headline news, it was determined that SARS had infected 8,400 people, killing 774 worldwide, with 33 probable U.S. cases and no deaths. After analyzing all the data from this outbreak, the WHO concluded that SARS is not spread easily through the air, but requires large respiratory droplets.

The Associated Press reported in October that fear over the possible return of SARS was so great in the United States that even if it didn't appear, the CDC expected emergency rooms to be swamped with suspected cases. They were concerned that doctors with limited SARS experience could confuse early SARS with the flu.

"Whether the virus comes back this winter or not, we will be dealing with SARS," said Dr. James Hughes, the director of the National Center for Infectious Diseases of the Centers for Disease Control and Prevention. "When people start showing up with respiratory diseases, physicians will be thinking of SARS. I can tell you we're more prepared than before,"

Hughes said. "I think the global community can handle SARS if it's handled appropriately. I think enough lessons have been learned" in the previous outbreak. Research on a vaccine and antiviral treatments were already underway, though tragically, they were stopped for lack of interest and funding, not knowing that a once in a lifetime pandemic would arise from a similar coronavirus sixteen years later. A fully tested SARS vaccine would have been of great use in 2020, as scientists began work on a SARS COV 2 vaccine.

As of February 2004, the outbreak still hadn't happened, with only three cases in Asia and none on the North American continent. But the new viral bug du jour was flu, not SARS. Hughes was wrong. By early 2004, SARS seemed like a distant memory.

We really don't know what stopped the SARS outbreak in spring 2003. It may simply have run its course. It seems likely that hand washing and isolation of infected individuals and travel restrictions helped, as the Times suggested in an editorial in early November 2003. But there was no direct evidence that the Times was right to conclude that "such tactics, buttressed by quarantines and restricted air travel, stopped the epidemic last time."

It clearly cost billions of dollars, and ironically, the Times editorial ended by reversing itself and cautioning the future use of aggressive tactics for SARS with a "recognition of the costs of any large-scale shutdown of normal activities."

But thanks to SARS hysteria, the apparatus was now in place for massive worldwide overreactions. If a disease died down, the health organizations and the media would take credit for its defeat without a true scientific study to prove they were right. If a disease seemed to get out of hand, the news media would continue to report it without ever acknowledging the way they—the media—were instantly altering the public's sense of risk.

In China, Zhong Nanshan, a scientist who had dealt with the first SARS outbreak, had a more practical plan. He urged people to avoid spitting in public and eating wild animals. Unfortunately, no one was listening to him either.

THE FEAR PROPHETS

God is with me, I shall not fear.

—Adon Olom prayer

Fear of the unknown and fear of death are primary fears, and they lead many people to religion. There is comfort to be found in the notion of a greater being who controls destiny. If a person makes peace with his or her god, then an inner serenity may be achieved.

Religion has worked well for many who struggle with deep questions that have no ready answers. If a patient suddenly receives a terminal diagnosis, her faith may sustain her through the harrowing process of dying.

Christianity and Judaism have taught that fearing God is the way to deal with the ultimate fear of death. We needn't fear death, instead we should revere God. A central passage in Jewish teachings states, "Raisheet chochmah yirat Adonoy—The beginning of wisdom is the awe of God" (Psalms 111:10).

In Christian theology, the principle of a loving God driving out the fear of the world is discussed in 1 John: "God is love . . . there is no fear in love. But perfect love drives out [worldly] fear, because fear has to do with punishment. The one who fears is not made perfect in love" (1 John 4:16b—18).

In the name of God throughout history, rather than preaching love and devotion, religious leaders have often used threats of retribution to get their followers to conform. (If you don't follow these rules, you may burn in hell.) Without doubt, religions can invoke fear as well as dispel it, but in times of tragedy and nervousness, many still turn to religion for comfort.

But religious leaders are not always equipped to handle day-today worries, superstitions, or unrealistic fears. In today's climate of fragmented and misguided information, an anxious alienated public may invoke spiritual platitudes that are difficult to apply to worldly concerns.

Priests, ministers, and rabbis are religion's go-to people, but they are not soothsayers. Nevertheless, the more nervous people become, worried out of proportion to real risks, frightened of hyped dangers, the more people present their clergy with questions that men of the cloth may not always be able to answer. God's representatives may grow weary, overwhelmed by their congregants' earthly panic.

A RABBI

About a month after Ephraim Azziz's operative date to remove the tiny cancer at the top of his lung, I received a phone call on Saturday evening, just after dusk. He had decided to call me at the conclusion of the Sabbath. His voice was still a hoarse whisper, not immediately recognizable.

"Thank you, doctor," he whispered. "You found it very early. Stage IA. These things usually kill you by the time they're found. But no lymph nodes. No spread. I'm clean. Some chemo and hopefully I'm done. Thank God."

I recalled showing his CT scan to my office mate, Dr. Madison, and how the disorganization at NYU before his needle biopsy had led him to have his surgery at the Memorial Sloan-Kettering Cancer Center. I hadn't expected to hear from him again after that.

"It's a good thing you came in when you did," I said, "and we decided not to wait on the CT scan. How are you feeling?"

"I'm weak. Very weak."

Two weeks later Azziz was back in my office examination room, covered with perspiration, breathing shallowly, and appearing fatigued. His hair had turned a new shade of gray, and his familiar tiny glasses were now crooked and greased. But a quick physical showed me that his vital signs were stable, his lungs were clear, and he had a normal temperature.

Despite his discomfort, it was clear to me that the purpose of his visit was not strictly medical—he was still under the direct care of the surgeon, but he was coming to me for reassurance.

He was in too much pain to sit straight on my blue office couch, so he half-sat, half-lounged.

"Let me tell you something, doctor," he said. "You are a man of science, not mysticism." His heavily accented voice added intrigue to his statement.

"I hope I am open-minded," I said.

"You know I am observant, a regular congregant at my synagogue. Do you know of the Rachamim? The mystical rabbis?"

"The Kabbalists," I said, and he smiled.

"Twelve years ago a Kabbalistic rabbi, as you call it, told me that I was supposed to die, but that God was going to have compassion on me. I've always remembered that. Now, you know it was two weeks before Rosh Hashanah, two weeks before I was to be inscribed in the book of life for the year, a week before you ordered the fateful CT scan, and I had a big fight with my wife. We came home from synagogue and she was upset. She said we had no life except the shul. We argued about it, and I went out again, but I had nowhere else to go, so I returned to the synagogue. It was the end of Shabbat, and I saw that there was a mystical rabbi there, famous from Israel, and there was a long line of people waiting to hear what he had to say. I stood at the end of the line, and by the time he got to me it was very dark outside. When he saw me, I could tell that he was startled. He told me that he was going to give me a new name, Mordecai."

"Why a new name?"

Azziz smiled slowly. "It is a tradition. It signifies a new life. Right away, he was telling me that I required a new identity. Sometimes things don't go right, he said. He said that he would write me a blessing on parchment and mail it to me from Israel."

"What happened?"

"When I got the results of the CT scan, I knew this was what he had meant. My wife said it was superstition, that these rabbis were just fortune-tellers, but I didn't agree. I telephoned the rabbi in Israel. I asked if he remembered me, and he did. I asked him what he saw, why he gave me another name. Here's what he said: 'In reincarnation, sometimes you come into this world with a sentence, something hanging over you from a previous life. But God gives you the means to undo that sentence, a medicine to treat it with. Your life has been spared,' the mystical rabbi told me. 'God will have compassion on you and there will be a new life for you, and everything will be okay.'

"I told him then the results of the CT scan, and he didn't seem surprised. He said again that I would be okay. The day of the operation, his letter arrived, with the parchment and the blessing."

We doctors had contributed to Azziz's well-being by discovering his cancer, then providing information that brought perspective and the hope appropriate with cancer that was found early. A doctor had swiftly removed the cancer with his scalpel and brought the chance for a cure.

But in the end Azziz was most comforted by the notion that both his illness and his recovery had been preordained, knowable only by the prescient powers of the mystical rabbis. Giving over control to their vision had helped him to make the difficult transition from apparent health to life-threatening illness in a short period of time. He'd been nervous and fearful, but he'd managed to cope.

Embracing this fateful view allowed him to take some of the responsibility away from cigarettes. But tobacco deserved no such pardon. The virile Marlboro Man images of smoking that corporate advertising had put over on us for so many years had a lot more to do with Azziz's cancer than the inevitability of fate.

Azziz was experiencing a fear that eclipsed even the usual fear of disease. Images of organ-wrenching cancer deaths have imbued it with a stigma that is difficult to face without becoming fatalistic. Azziz's fear was out of proportion to the risk of even cancer, because of the Internet and media hype and misinformation that had conditioned him. Cancer info-bites petrify people. It was unfortunate that the only relief for Azziz was to be found in the reassuring words and miraculous vision of an all-knowing mystic. In a world of such isolation, these were the only tools Azziz could find to help him regain his purpose.

TWO PRIESTS

Two priests were patients in my practice for several years, though I didn't connect them in my mind. They both served as chaplains to the New York City Fire Department, but they rarely met at FDNY functions, and not once in my office waiting room. They were different kinds of men. Father Mychal Judge, a Franciscan friar who lacked a parish, was a public figure who provided succor to firefighters as well as to everyone from the homeless to the famous. He served on soup lines and was also a regular guest at both Gracie Mansion and the Clinton White House.

A visit to my medical office from Judge meant a waiting room confessional involving Judge and several of my patients. Getting him to confide in me wasn't as easy. He accepted the samples of blood pressure medications I gave him, but he didn't seem concerned for his health, only for the health of others. Judge said he was not afraid of getting sick or of dying.

Father "John Henderson," on the other hand, was a private man. He too had high blood pressure and accepted samples, but beyond this, the similarity to Judge seemed to end. Henderson had his own parish in the heart of working man's Brooklyn; he was usually to be found in his study reading, or in the rectory, or meeting with his congregants. He was involved with the fire department only when they called him, sometimes when Judge was out of town visiting various dignitaries, including the Clintons.

Judge was not a favorite of Cardinal O'Connor, because Judge frequently upstaged him—and there was the time when a bereaved widow insisted that Friar Judge rather than the cardinal perform the funeral services for her husband at St. Patrick's Cathedral.

When Judge required sudden surgery for abdominal pain, he didn't show fear or worry, even after the surgeon took out a perfectly normal gall bladder and left in a festering part of the colon. Judge went through the second surgery without placing blame. He said he would ask God to forgive the surgeon's mistake. Judge was a clear example of how a person could stay centered, not allowing his perspective to be altered by panic.

I was hoping that the day would come when I could reassure Father Judge the way he did others, but he didn't require it from me. When his insurance lapsed, he didn't come to my office for many months, not wanting to accept my charity. When he died suddenly in the World Trade Center rescue operations on 9/11, it was with courage rather than fear.

Surely Judge, if he had lived, would have remained a go-to person in our hysteria-ridden times. While he was alive, he was a sponge for others' fear as well as a role model for courage.

THE FEAR COUNSELOR

After Father Judge died, Father Henderson became very busy. He was compelled to ignore his own parish, taking Judge's prominent place amid complaints that this unassuming padre was no Father Judge. Henderson was the first to admit it.

But he had his own style, and he worked tirelessly through the evenings and late into the night calming the shocked and bereaved survivors of 9/11, the families, and the firefighters. He officiated at many of the funerals, but because of his halting speech, it was lost on many who attended just how eloquent his sermons were.

Henderson lacked Judge's flamboyance, but not his purpose, and his faith salved many psychic wounds. He helped people who were frightened to retain control of their lives by continuing to work and care for their families. He encouraged people to stay within their usual patterns of living.

I think that Henderson expected the complaints to slow down, as people readjusted to the post-9/11 world. Instead, with a continued high volume of calls he began to grow more and more uneasy. He no longer slept well at night, and he frequently forgot to shave. He also began to question the nature of the complaints. People were worried about another attack, they were worried about toxins in the air, they were worried about every bug du jour, and they were worried about their children's future. All this was understandable, but Henderson recognized that his role was transforming into that of a therapist. People were consulting him and needing to speak to him about worries that had little to do with his being a priest.

One night in April 2003, he returned home to his empty silent room at the church rectory at 2 A.M., and as he lay in his bed sleeplessly thinking, an old regret pained him—he didn't have a family. His life was becoming a collection of the frets and fears of his congregants.

The next day, Henderson appeared in my office in the late afternoon without an appointment, just before my staff was about to leave for the day. Seeing one of her favorite patients arrive bundled in an overcoat that was too heavy for the mild spring weather, my office nurse quickly ushered him into one of the examining rooms.

Henderson didn't speak. His blood pressure was normal and his physical exam and EKG unremarkable. I told him to dress, and he followed me to my pale blue brick consultation room. Sitting on the couch across from me, he stared out the window toward the Empire State Building.

"What's the matter, John?" I asked. "Why are you here?"

When he looked at me, he began wringing his hands until they reddened.

"I haven't been sleeping," he said slowly.

"Why not?"

"I'm out all evening. The whole city is in a panic. They're geared up for something, but they don't know what it is or when it's going to come. They can't seem to calm down."

I wasn't sure whether he was referring to a specific scare. SARS was just becoming "newsworthy" at the time of this office visit but wasn't yet in full swing.

"Who is afraid?"

"It's everyone. Not just the orphans and widows, not just the firefighters or their families. People stop me on the street: 'Father, can you help me?' 'Father, can I please talk to you?'"

"What do you tell them?"

He smiled. We had known each other for many years, and he was comfortable with my bluntness.

"Come on, Doc. You know what I tell them. I tell them to have faith. I tell them that everything is beyond their control, that they have to give their worries over to a merciful creator."

"Does this help them?"

"It helps them. But does it help me?! I absorb this, and then I can't sleep at night. I have my faith but it's not always enough. And what are they worried about? They worry about bombs and threats that haven't happened and may never happen. My parishioners, the firefighters, their families, their doubts overwhelm me. What am I supposed to do?"

This was more than he had said to me in all the years I'd known him. I'd met Father Henderson in 1993 following the stroke of his brother, Thomas, an accomplished botanist. I'd cared for Thomas through a blood clot in his leg, two bouts of pneumonia, and ultimately, the pancreatic cancer in 1999 that took his life. John brought his brother in his wheelchair to most of his doctors' visits. At home, he injected him with morphine to control the pain. In the end, he helped his brother accept his death.

Even in the period of grief following this, John didn't appear as somber as he did now.

"Are you depressed?" I asked.

He thought about it. "No."

"Anxious, overwhelmed?"

"That's more like it."

"I can give you a mild tranquilizer at night called Klonopin that will help you break the cycle. You might be a little sleepy from it in the morning, but a cup of coffee will counter that."

He nodded that he would take the prescription.

"Father, do you know what you're afraid of?"

Henderson smiled.

"I'm not afraid of dying. Every day I pray for acceptance of my fate. But most who turn to me for help are afraid of dying. I think that's where their vulnerability comes from. People are in a panic every day now, they feel out of control. Their specific fears may be made up by the politicians or the TV, but it feels real to them. And I think I am absorbing this worry. I absorb it by osmosis, and it becomes difficult for me to control."

"What do you do?"

He sighed. "Back when I was a kid and something would frighten me, I remember coming home alone at night and seeing my father sitting in the warm kitchen, reading his paper and drinking his tea the way he did every night to relax. He would just wink at me, and I would be reassured. The apprehension would be gone, knowing he was the last stop for me."

"What do you do now?"

"I came here to see you today."

Father Henderson stood up then, and we shook hands.

"Thanks, Doc," he said.

"I want to see you again in two weeks," I said. "And don't reschedule."

John wouldn't go for psychotherapy, but he continued to come to see me in this manner, over several weeks. He rarely needed to take the Klonopin, and after five visits, he said he felt better.

I was flattered, realizing that the earthly comfort John was seeking was simply to know that he could confide in someone. In my office, where the staff treated him warmly, he could be diverted from the chaos of war anxiety. He had absorbed the irrational fears until he was radioactive with them.

Father Henderson and his enduring faith had always provided a haven for others from fear. His parish was for many their only consolation. When he was overwhelmed, however, my office was his haven, like the kitchen of his childhood. I served as a reminder of the comfort his father had provided on those days when a son came home frightened on a dark night.

THE FEAR PROPHET

Of all the speakers at the fear conference at the New School so long ago in February 2004, Tom Pyszczynski, the originator of terror management theory, was the most unassuming, the most soft-spoken, and yet his central idea has stayed with me most vividly over all these years. His long white hair flowing to his shoulders like a postmodern wizard's, he spoke about all fear emanating from a central fear of death.

If this is true for animals, it is truer for humans, who, like our animal predecessors, can be instinctively petrified of death and, in addition, be petrified by the contemplation of death. Pyszczynski, a psychologist, saw the basic human need to sublimate this central fear in culture and society. But when the society we build for ourselves begins to deteriorate, as this one has, it no longer absorbs our fears. Our safety net of information and communicated risk is suspect. We are frightened for our lives beyond any realistic danger by those we've appointed as our protectors.

For many, faith is the only consolation. Faith takes the worry away and transfers it to a higher Being who is controlling the world. Any sense of control we have is illusory. And yet, we obsess on control and fear its loss.

These days our culture of worry is a growing weed that feeds on manufactured as well as real pandemic dangers and threatens to become its own cult. Traditional religion may not be a match for it. Religion works best when it engages the unanswerable questions, where faith is paramount in coping with the uncertainty of death. But religion has become overloaded with today's obsessive worry and no longer serves as a reliable cure for fear.

Of course if anyone can save us from ourselves, God can.

IS THERE A CURE
FOR FEAR?

I liberated myself from the fear by creating these works.
Their creation had the purpose of healing myself.

—Japanese artist Yayoi Kusama in an interview

Nor should we forget that courage is contagious,
that it overcomes the silence and fear that estrange people
from one another.

—Paul Rogat Loeb, *The Impossible Will Take a Little While:
A Citizen's Guide to Hope in a Time of Fear*

If fear is no longer protective, if it has been transformed from an adaptive tool into a symptomatic illness, then we have to find a way to cure it.

The spread of fear has reached epidemic proportions. The national media broadcast threats and warp our perspective. The sense of immediate danger is highly contagious.

To slow the spread of fear, it is necessary to "vaccinate" with reason those who aren't yet afflicted. A population that is slow to react hysterically helps contain fear. But lasting immunity to the epidemic of fear is difficult to attain. The biochemistry is built into our brains, waiting to be triggered.

Once fear has been elicited, it is stored deep in the emotional memory, ready to emerge whenever the so-called danger recurs.

In early 2004, months before she broke her leg, my daughter, Rebecca, was taking a bath. She was almost three years old at the time, the time when the brain circuitry completes its wiring of the "safety center" in the prefrontal cortex. She had never before experienced the bubble effect, and when the Jacuzzi device in the tub turned on automatically, I was on the other side of the apartment. By the time I rushed back to the tub, she was petrified, standing straight up, bright red from crying.

For months afterward, she was afraid to take a bath at all. I tried to appeal to her newly working brain center to suppress the fear that this tub would always bring the scary bubbles, but the fear response was too strong.

This is the reality that we encounter in America in the twenty-first century. Once alerted, once afraid, it is hard to turn the switch back to the off position. This was certainly true for the COVID pandemic in 2020—the problem, which was bad enough, was magnified enormously through fear terms such as "second wave" and "lockdown" and "mandate." Lost was the fact that by late summer the virus appeared to be burning itself out as the new case and death and hospitalization rates dropped and the immunity against the virus, especially in populations most at risk, rose.

The news signals danger, and we instantly fear it. A person living in a small town in the heartland who watches cable news may experience the fear almost as much as a big-city dweller who has an infinitely greater risk of witnessing terrorism up close.

Of course, one simple cure is to turn off the TV.

A NEW EQUATION

There is no standard treatment for fear in part because the symptoms vary from one person to the next. A person may feel destined to a certain bad outcome and have a greater sense of foreboding because of a certain family tendency. Some people more easily trigger a fight-or-flight flood of hormones than others.

My wife's mother has a severe case of multiple sclerosis and has been confined to a wheelchair for almost forty years. Over the years my wife has confided in me her fear that she could be next. Every time she brings up her perception that MS could be in her future, I try to counter it with the bald statistic that only 4 percent of first-degree relatives are at risk for the disease. "There is a 96 percent chance that you won't get it," I say, but for my wife, as for many others, the perception rests with the 4 percent.

Empathy for her mother and a natural tendency to personalize her experience create the fear and the conviction. What finally overcame her emotions and concernswas the completely negative MRI of the brain she had.

Recurrent or unremitting fear has the same effect on the human body that running an engine persistently at 80 to 100 mph has on a car. For a person who is always on the alert, who suffers from a too easily triggered and sustained fight-or-flight response, the result is a burned-out body. Many illnesses are more likely to occur as a result, including heart disease, cancer, stroke, and depression. What we have most to fear are not the exotic diseases that scare us, but the ordinary killers such as heart attacks that develop as a result of our unremitting worries.

We are scaring ourselves about the wrong things in a way that is clearly a terrorist's delight. (We do much of their work for them.)

We need to be reeducated as a prerequisite to healing fear. We tend to overpersonalize much of the information we receive. We need a new sense of proportion to correct this.

THE FEAR VACCINE

How calm can a patient be these days?

Can we be reeducated not to trigger our fear, or will there instead be a simple pill that cures us all, or a fear vaccine? Oh, how we love our miracle cures.

In a study by Jonathan Kipnis et al. in Israel published in the Proceedings of the National Academy of Sciences in May 2004, the authors gave an immunological vaccine to mice in whom they had previously induced psychosis. This chemical cocktail bolstered the nerve cells, and the state of panic and paranoia ended. The mice were once again able to perform their usual tasks.

The implication of these results is that immunological "vaccines" could have a role in reversing fear. If this supposition proves to be true, instead of learning healthier contexts, we will be able to obscure our hysteria with immunology.

Fear vaccines raise similar ethical issues as medicating an entire society with beta blockers or other antianxiety treatments. As our fear grows, the reach for soothing salves is typical of American consumerism. It is one thing to employ sophisticated technologies to heal the sick, to control psychosis, or to bolster a nerve fiber in a troubled brain. It is another to bottle the latest preventative and market it widely to treat all fear.

A CHEMICAL CURE

As I discussed earlier in the book, Joe Ledoux has determined that fear memory in rats is deeply rooted and predominates over other types of rational memory. Ledoux showed that when rats are given the medicine anisomycin, their fear memory is blocked. Based on these results, Roger Pitman, a professor of psychiatry at Harvard, theorized that administering the beta-blocker drug propranolol can also block fear memory and blunt the fight-or-flight response.

Pitman and his group looked at the effects of giving propranolol within six hours of a traumatic event (mostly car accidents). One month afterward, he was able to determine a significantly lower incidence of posttraumatic stress disorder than in the control group. Larry Cahill, at the Irvine, California, memory center, also tested the effects of propranolol on humans and found that it prevented people from recalling a gory story better than a bland story.

But blunting fear memory with medication is not the same thing as retraining the brain. It seems fruitless to provoke fear unnecessarily and then have to develop drugs to reverse it.

Descartes argued in The Passions of the Soul that "all the harm they [the passions] can cause consists in their fortifying and conserving those thoughts more than is needed, or in fortifying and conserving others which ought not to be fixed there." Descartes was referring to the damaging effects of negative emotions. He felt we could become obsessed with our own dark thoughts. Almost four hundred years later, we as a society may be even more susceptible to these fears.

I described the work of Rachel Yehuda earlier in this book. Dr. Yehuda has concluded that PTSD is too much in vogue in a way that harms us. Many people who simply read or hear about a trauma think they are suffering from it. Unnecessary anguish is often an overreaction to another person's trauma. We stimulate our voyeuristic suffering and then find we may have to medicate ourselves to cool down.

Our fear-for-profit culture is too ready to latch on to the next drug to regulate us. Imagine the drug company ears pricking up to this new role for beta blockers. The new drug company TV ad is sure to be, "Are you stressed? Do you experience posttraumatic stress? Try this . . ."

Pills become our crutches. Drug ads and our popular culture teach us to treat our cholesterol with pills rather than diet; our obesity responds to amphetamines rather than exercise; we clog our coronary arteries thoughtlessly and then "Roto-Rooter" them open. We come to depend on these treatments. We are afraid to do without them.

This medication dependency is not that dissimilar to many of our other product dependencies. We deplete the world's oil reserves built from millions of years of organic decay, and pollute the skies with our engines. All because we are afraid of the dark, or the cold, or the heat. We lead temperature-controlled, environment-controlled lives. We are afraid of aging, so we plastic-surgerize our bodies to the best approximation of youth that we can obtain.

All this environmental control stems back to our ultimate fear of death. We hide behind the illusion provided by technology, but ultimately, fear of death seeps through. True culture, art, philosophy, and science provide better depositories for human angst. Religious faith can help us to cope with our fear of death, but it can also be misappropriated by superstitious fears, as demonstrated in the last chapter.

In twenty-first-century America, we worship the god of wealth. We medicate ourselves with the emotional anesthesia of materialism, but our fears seep in and overtake us anyway.

THE POLITICS OF UNHEALING

Preventing fear means developing a strategy that emphasizes that you aren't going to get a disease just because someone else a thousand miles away from you has gotten it. Preventing fear means learning that if there are holes in the so-called safety net, it matters only if the threat itself is real.

Instead, we are too often warned about things that don't threaten us directly, while at the same time, ho-hum killers that can really get us—the overuse of Tylenol and Advil, for example—are being ignored in our medicine cabinets.

Treating fear means gaining a real perspective on danger, redirecting our attention to those diseases that really can kill us, and developing a well-reasoned response to these real threats. COVID-19 is a real risk, real threat, but so are all the other health threats—mental and physical—that mushroom while we fixate on COVID.

HEALING HYPOCHONDRIACS

Living in a climate of fear, we are becoming a society of hypochondriacs. Many people worry excessively over the slightest symptom, often convinced that they are sick. This summer I treated an army of patients (most of them by televisits) who were convinced they had COVID, and the vast majority of them didn't. According to the American Psychiatric Association, a hypochondriac is a patient who fears that he has a serious disease for at least six months despite doctors' attempts to reassure him that he is healthy. This definition is beginning to apply to more and more of us.

The ancient Greeks coined the term hypochondria to refer to melancholy symptoms that they associated with certain organs in men beneath the rib cage. In women, symptoms of "hysteria" were related to problems with the womb. It wasn't until the seventeenth century that physicians began to realize that these fears originated in the brain.

At the end of the twentieth century, when Ledoux and others began to map our fear circuitry, they uncovered the neural network of fear that involves the body's organs as well as the brain. So the Greeks weren't completely wrong in their beliefs.

Can the process that leads to hypochondria be reversed? Dr. Arthur Barsky of Harvard published a study in the Journal of the American Medical Association looking at the effect of teaching hypochondriacs to pay less attention to their symptoms. The results were analyzed at six-month and one-year intervals. Patients were taught to suspend their usual ways of responding to their fears, which included searching the Internet, taking their own vital signs, and scheduling excessive doctors' appointments. Doctors were coached to see their patients only for regular appointments and not to schedule tests as a knee-jerk response.

In this JAMA study, Barsky observed that patients receiving this therapy "had significantly lower levels of hypochondriacal symptoms, beliefs, and attitudes . . . and health-related anxiety. They also had significantly less impairment of . . . activities of daily living."

In my medical practice, I have observed that many patients who aren't the full-blown hypochondriacs of Barsky's study share a fear of death and disease that often overwhelms their ability to reason. I have found that many of these patients do better when they keep a sense of control rather than have strict limits imposed on them. Over time, these limits may not decrease fear as Barsky's study suggests. I have found that giving over this control to a physician is comforting only when a patient feels that this is her choice. Many patients who insist on reviewing their blood test results become even more apprehensive if a doctor tries to withhold these results. Deconditioning may be somewhat helpful, but primitive emotions like fear will find new outlets unless dealt with on a deeper level.

I had a visit from my patient "Zeke," whose father had died from an abdominal aneurysm. All of Zeke's siblings were suddenly worried that they too had aneurysms. I reassured Zeke that it didn't tend to run in families, which helped some. I listened to Zeke's abdomen and found no noisy bruits to correspond to an aneurysm, which reassured him further. Ultimately it took an abdominal ultrasound to completely reassure him that he didn't have an aneurysm, a test that Barsky might have considered excessive, but it did the trick. Though Zeke wasn't a textbook hypochondriac, his fears were extended by grieving in a way that required extra reassurance.

Hypochondriacs are people with an excessive fear of death translated into a multitude of neuroses about life. We all have these fears, but for some they are more overwhelming than for others. And illness isn't the only direct metaphor for death. Legal hypochondriacs are those of us who are always calling our lawyers and worrying about the possibility of suing or being sued—I am one of those people for whom a lawsuit represents death. Luckily, my lawyer is a close friend and doesn't charge for my calls.

My wife is a financial hypochondriac, which means that she worries that everything will cost more money than we have. For her, bankruptcy means death. Our accountant handles my wife's concerns but then sends us large bills for the service, which worries her further.

Mostly, we are becoming a society of hypochondriacs, not just for medical reasons, but because of preoccupations in all aspects of our lives. We build elaborate safety nets for the wrong things, and then we panic when these nets are found to be ineffective.

Healing this rampant fear means all of us becoming our own filters for information, not simply parroting what we hear on TV. We need to be deconditioned, decontaminated, and decompressed from the high-pressure misinformation that is being shot into our brains. Once purged, once healed of our programmed fears, and with the help of knowledgeable go-to people who really care about us, we can reappraise the safety of our lives.

Unfortunately, the coronavirus pandemic may not be the best time to learn to overcome our fears completely, though it is certainly the time to learn to control them better.

ANTIDOTES FOR FEAR

MACBETH: Canst thou not minister to a mind diseas'd,
                 Pluck from the memory a rooted sorrow,
                 Raze out the rooted troubles of the brain,
                 And with some sweet oblivious antidote,
                 Cleanse the stuff'd bosom of that perilous stuff
                 Which weighs upon the heart?

DOCTOR: Therein the patient
                 Must minister to himself.

For years, I have tried to help people handle their disease fears without knowing if I am succeeding or not. In studying the fear circuitry of the brain, I have now come to appreciate that teaching might not automatically lead to learning. Fear is a deep-rooted emotion, difficult for the brain to control. Sometimes its triggering can't be avoided. My daughter's early life experience with the bubbles as well as with her broken leg educated me that if fear is unlearned, it is because a new emotion replaces it. This healing occurs at its own rate of speed and a parent, or a doctor, has little control over it.

Fear is an important factor in illness that hasn't been well accounted for. Physical, as well as psychological, breakdown occurs at an accelerated rate under the pressure of persistent fear. Science now has the brain-mapping and chemical-testing prowess to help determine exactly how this happens. Unfortunately, we still have a long way to go before we stop unnecessarily triggering the fear circuit in the first place.

Once triggered, fear is personal and too often intractable. People may fear anyone or anything they perceive as alien, from terrorism to atheism to crime to disease to noise. But all of this fear of the "other" ultimately stems from a fear of obliteration or death.

To conquer fear we must return it to its primitive place as an instinct. We must stop overpersonalizing it. We must regain our footing with regular sleep, regular meals, regular entertainment, regular exercise, and regular work. We must resist those who choose the wrong danger, hype the need to respond, and then bungle the response—making the threat seem even more real. We must replace our unreal fears with real courage.

CURING A MIDLIFE CRISIS

One patient revealed to me how fear could be healed.

"Joel Enrand" was suffering from depression, weight gain, high cholesterol, and elevated blood pressure. Many studies in the medical literature predicted these conditions would get worse if left untreated.

Mr. Enrand was a police detective and had endured the stress of many undercover investigations. He had just turned forty, and he planned to retire from the police force in five more years with a good pension. In the meantime, he was finding his job more and more difficult to perform. He had been married for almost twenty years and his son was a young teenager.

His mental deterioration may have been gradual, but it was during an office visit in midsummer that I noticed the change. Formerly a clap-you-on-the-shoulder type, on this visit he was timid, speaking too softly to be understood. His curly hair had become an untrimmed shrub, and the office scale recorded a thirty-pound weight gain on his muscular frame. I noticed that his roughskinned face and neck had reddened, which may have been from the direct effect of stress hormones.

"I can't sleep," he said.

"Why not?"

"Things aren't so good with my wife."

He described a home situation that had devolved into screaming fights in front of his son. She yelled at him for coming home late. He yelled at her for yelling. She accused him of being with other women. He denied it. My instinct was to believe him.

I suggested that he see a therapist for the anxiety. He refused, saying he wasn't crazy.

I offered to treat his anxiety with Valium and Prozac. For his rising blood pressure I had in mind Lisinopril, a pill that dilates arteries, and for his high cholesterol I offered the ever-popular Lipitor (my patient looked nothing like the smiling healthy people advertising cholesterol drugs on TV). Once his blood pressure was under control, I could add an amphetamine for his obesity, and if his blood pressure rose as a result, I would increase the blood pressure medicine to compensate.

He showed little interest in these suggestions.

I was hoping that he would at least look to me to help him through this period of stress. Instead, he stopped coming to his appointments altogether, and when I called him on the phone, it was apparent that though he was suffering miserably, he wasn't about to listen to me.

I finally managed to convince him to see me one more time, and knowing this might be his final visit, I knew I had to rethink my approach. Trying to force him onto medications only underlined his deterioration, offered him a crutch, and made him identify himself as sick. Perhaps he felt that if he admitted to this weakness, he might break down altogether.

During our next meeting, Enrand admitted that he had an overriding fear of losing everything—his health, his job, his family. Most of all, with paralyzing middle-of-the-night bouts of sleepless fright, he was afraid he was losing his mind.

"You're not crazy," I said, and on hearing this, the tiny muscles around his eyes relaxed.

I realized then that fear was his illness, not the high blood pressure, obesity, or cholesterol that developed as a result. Perhaps his apprehension would diminish if he was able to continue his life and not lose what he feared losing.

I watched him, offering nothing. I had no choice now but to allow him to remain in control, as bit by bit he reinstituted his disciplines. He continued working. He refused couples therapy, but I think he was reassured by the simple fact that his wife stayed with him.

He finally asked me for Valium to take in the middle of the night, as his one medicine to break the cycle of worry. He began to admit he was depressed, but he still wouldn't take an antidepressant. I think he took pride in fighting depression without pills, and used this pride to help rebuild his self-esteem.

In the mornings, he willed himself to jog three miles before work. He ate two to three meals per day but didn't binge. He allowed himself two cigars per week, calling them his one vice.

He missed many doctor's visits but called me every few weeks. When he did come, I examined him and recorded his improving blood pressure. I suspected I was recording the physiological effects of a diminishing fear. Mostly I just sat and talked with him in my consultation room.

There was a correlation between his returning well-being and his personal grooming. On the same visit where I noticed his hair was combed and trimmed in the old fashion, he told me that things were better between him and his wife; he was no longer sleeping on the couch; he was no longer staying out late at night.

He began to enjoy his cronies at work again, the brief interludes of clowning and kidding. He talked with enthusiasm about tracking down the evidence that the DA needed to convict a notorious child molester.

Six months after reluctantly agreeing to Enrand's method, I measured his blood pressure and discovered it was back down to normal without treatment. My office scale indicated that he had lost thirty pounds over that time. His cholesterol was back below 190. Now he was sleeping through the night without Valium.

Looking at him sitting relaxed on the couch across from me, I knew that I would be seeing him less often, whether I scheduled appointments for him or not.

"My courage is back, Doc," he said.

He looked at me and I was glad to see the return of his purposeful expression.

"Things were happening to me. I latched onto the worry. I could feel it, like it was real. It gripped me, and it grew."

"But you fought it?"

"Just by sticking to routines, rituals, they replaced the doubts little by little. When I saw I was getting my life back, I started to enjoy the routines."

Enrand hesitated. "Most importantly," he said, "I'd always wanted to be a dad, and I loved my son more than anything, and I knew I was responsible for him. He needed me, and I grew stronger by refusing to let go of him."

Now that Enrand had passed through his midlife crisis, we both realized that he'd been doing the doctoring. He'd learned to treat—not physical illness—but fear.

In the end, his plan was far better than mine. He lost weight, his blood pressure and cholesterol went down, and his spirits and his marriage improved. I suspected that his stress hormones, which were responsible for his high blood pressure and anxiety, were now diminished.

I was merely a witness to this change, though I learned a big lesson. Committing him to three or four new pills might have led me to the erroneous conclusion that the medicines were responsible for his improvement, rather than his courage. And once started, how would I have known when to stop them?

BIRD FLU AND
SWINE FLU

On November 20, 2005, Dr. Anthony Fauci, director of the NIH's National Institutes of Allergy and Infectious Diseases was among a panel of experts interviewed on NBC's Meet the Press by moderator Tim Russert.

Mr. Russert: "Dr. Fauci, how do you explain this to people, that we're here talking about this possibility of a pandemic flu? One, how much of a possibility is it, in your mind? Two, how fearful should people be?"

Dr. Fauci: "I think it's important to put into context a pandemic flu in general. . . . We had the worst-case scenario in 1918 with . . . 50 million people dead. . . . If you look at the situation in 1968, it was really dramatically different. It was still a pandemic . . . but relatively speaking, it was rather mild. . . . Sooner or later, the way viruses evolve, we're gonna get another pandemic. It could be a couple years from now; it could be 15 or 20 years from now. If it doesn't happen, that doesn't mean that preparedness went to waste, because sooner or later it's going to happen."

WHAT IS BIRD FLU?

All bird flus are influenza A. Influenza A is primarily a respiratory virus in humans, causing coughing, congestion, sore throat, muscle aches, fatigue, and fever in most species it infects.

The 2006 strain (also called the H5N1 virus) surfaced in Hong Kong in the late 1990s, although it might have been around for four decades previous to this. It was mostly been affecting Asian poultry. When tested in the laboratory, it was found to be quite deadly, killing ten out of ten chick embryos against which it was tested. It was difficult to tell how many birds it killed in Asia, though, because millions of birds were killed by humans to prevent its spread. As soon as one chicken developed symptoms, it was killed along with all the chickens that may have come in contact with it.

It appeared to be quite deadly to humans as well, although in Hong Kong in 1997 many humans reportedly developed antibodies to the virus and did not get sick. There was concern that if the virus mutated, it could cause a pandemic because we did not have built-up immunity to it. This mutation could occur either at random or if the virus mixed its DNA with a human flu virus inside a pig or a human. But it was also quite possible (in fact much more likely) that it would never mutate at all in a major way or even if it did, the mutated virus would result in a much less severe illness in humans.

WHAT IS INFLUENZA?

Influenza is a virus. Unlike bacteria, which are single cells, a virus is not a full cell and cannot reproduce on its own. To reproduce, a virus infects a cell and uses the resources of that cell. Essentially, a virus is just a sack of genetic material enclosed by a protein envelope. Viruses don't even fit the definition of "alive," though most scientists agree that they are.

There are two types of viruses: DNA (deoxyribonucleic acid) and RNA (ribonucleic acid). Influenza is a single stranded RNA virus. Influenza comes in two main varieties: A and B. (It also comes in a C, which rarely causes illness.) Influenza A viruses are found in many different animals, including ducks, chickens, pigs, whales, horses, and seals. Influenza B viruses circulate widely only among humans and generally do not make us as sick as influenza A does.

Influenza A viruses are divided into subtypes based on two bumpy proteins on the surface of the virus: the hemagglutinin (H) and the neuraminidase (N). These two identifying proteins are why the current bird flu is referred to as H5N1. There are 16 different hemagglutinin subtypes and 9 different neuraminidase subtypes, all of which have been found among influenza A viruses in wild birds. H5 and H7 subtypes include all the current pathogenic strains.

HOW DOES INFLUENZA SPREAD AND WHAT COMPLICATIONS DOES IT CAUSE?

Influenza is spread by airborne droplets and is inhaled into the respiratory tract. It incubates in the body from one to four days before a person feels ill. Complications tend to occur in the very young, in the elderly, and in patients with chronic cardiopulmonary diseases. The major complication of flu is pneumonia from influenza itself, or bacterial pneumonia from pneumococcus or haemophilus.

H5N1

In 1997, an apparent new strain of influenza A broke out in Hong Kong in birds (it was discovered later that this strain may have dated back to the 1950s). At the time, local officials thought they had gotten it under control. But when it reappeared a few years later, this strain (H5N1), perhaps because it was continuing to mutate, spread more quickly and over a larger geographical area than most previous influenzas, decimating the feathered population in its wake. Millions of birds were killed. Scientists became worried about their inability to prepare for and manage, let alone eliminate, this threat. For chickens, this was easily the most terrifying thing to happen since Colonel Sanders opened for business. For humans, the risk remained mostly theoretical.

The H5N1 virus remained primarily an avian virus, and the population it has decimated is primarily poultry. At least three hundred people died, which was inarguably tragic, but the total number was very small compared to the toll of almost every other disease currently taking human lives.

But you could also see why, if the virus were ever to affect humans in the same way it did birds, it could be calamitous. Everyone who followed this story needed to understand both sides of the discussion. The fear surrounding avian flu came not from what was actually happening, but from what-if scenarios.

People worried: What if the disease became a human virus that spread just as quickly among humans and remained just as deadly? It was an important question, but for nonscientists it was easy to become confused about how likely the bird flu pandemic scenario was. We needed to be in awe of the potential for damage, while learning to understand why the likelihood of the worst case coming to pass was awfully low. For one thing, H5 or H7 for that matter, were not the type of hemagglutinin proteins that had ever mutated in the direction of easy human to human transmission. And as the years passed without sustained human outbreaks, it became clear that this was the case for H5N1 too. We had spent a lot of time worrying unnecessarily.

THE SPANISH FLU

In early March 1918, before significant numbers of American GIs had even arrived in the killing fields of Europe, a few soldiers at Camp Funston, Kansas, came down with the flu. Within days, hundreds of soldiers at the camp were sick. At the time, and for many years afterward, no one knew where this new strain of the influenza virus had come from, and the medical personnel at Camp Funston couldn't have imagined where it would go.

Still, it didn't catch the American medical establishment completely by surprise. In past wars, the number of dead due to disease compared to or surpassed the number killed in combat, and most military doctors expected this war to be no different. It was unimaginable that the day might come when fighting epidemic disease wasn't synonymous with fighting a war.

In fact, during the war, epidemics of microorganisms that incubated among groups of closely packed, unhealthy soldiers eventually affected the civilian population. In addition, doctors and nurses called to the front to treat combat injuries were obviously no longer available to attend to epidemic sufferers, military or civilian.

War planners understood that the likeliest candidate for an epidemic was bacterial pneumonia, because in that era it was the leading cause of death in America every year. But germ theory was just gaining acceptance, and scientists still didn't completely understand viruses. In fact, bacteria also played a role with Spanish flu, as bacterial pneumonia and sinus infections were common secondary complications and leading causes of death brought on by the H1N1 Spanish flu virus.

This H1N1 strain is frequently referred to as the Spanish flu even though it neither started in Spain nor peaked there, although Spain did have one of the worst early outbreaks. The Spanish discussed this strange flu more extensively than in many other cultures. They had not been drawn into the war, so they weren't censoring their news to manipulate public morale and were able to devote more of their national debate to the topic.

The Spanish flu virus emerged in 1918 the same way all variations on the influenza virus do. The flu virus spread from person to person, probably in very cramped quarters, via airborne respiratory secretions, the familiar coughing and sneezing of any respiratory infection. The first wave of infections was relatively mild. By August, the H1N1 strain appeared to have become more lethal. It has been speculated that after passing once around the world, it must have mutated into something more effective at reaching deep into the lungs of its victims, perhaps turning the immune systems of young and healthy victims against them as they choked on copious secretions. Or perhaps it affected younger patients more severely because they selectively lacked immunity to an older, related virus from the prior century. In any case, the virus spread more and more quickly, zooming around the globe again, this time as a true pandemic. Dr. Jeffrey Taubenberger, famed flu researcher, has suggested that the fall outbreak could have been due to a different, more deadly, flu virus. To take just one example of its fury in an American military facility, one reported infection at Camp Devens, Massachusetts, became 6,674 cases in only six days. By 1919, the flu had killed at least 500,000 Americans and perhaps as many as 50 million or more across the rest of the world, wreaking the most havoc in India, where it killed 17 million.

The Spanish flu was easily the most destructive influenza outbreak in history. As has been widely reported, more U.S. soldiers died from the Spanish flu during World War I than from war injuries.

FLU ORIGINS

It is far more likely that the Spanish flu actually began in Asia or India rather than among the poultry population in Kansas. In the 1990s, the H1N1 virus, which has been preserved from several victims, was studied in the laboratory, and determinations were made about what had happened back in 1918. H1N1 most likely started out in waterfowl, like most influenza A viruses, and then infected poultry before mutating to a form that could easily infect humans. There is no record of a large outbreak in birds, and it is reasonable to conclude that this virus, so deadly to humans after it mutated, was not that deadly to birds beforehand.

Poultry, including chickens and turkeys, are bred for all sorts of characteristics, mostly related to the amount and quality of meat each bird can produce. Wildfowl, however, are concerned only with survival, and as one might expect, they are more resistant to diseases, including influenza infections, than their domestic counterparts.

All birds are susceptible to avian influenza, although some species are more resistant than others. In birds, different strains of flu can cause any range of symptoms, from mild illness to a highly contagious and rapidly fatal disease. Strains with a sudden onset, severe illness, and rapid death are called highly pathogenic avian influenza.

Migratory waterfowl, especially ducks, are the natural reservoir of the avian influenza virus. They harbor the viruses in their GI tract and spread it through their feces.

Many influenza epidemics among birds occur when ducks or geese with a new strain of virus come into contact with poultry. Domestic poultry are carefully monitored for influenza, even the mildest cases, because their lower tolerance means one infection can quickly become a highly fatal epidemic. This is especially true for H5 or H7 varieties of avian flu, which tend to be the most deadly among birds.

If a mutation occurs to allow an influenza A we've been exposed to before to pass among humans, it can become our yearly flu strain. (Influenza B occurs natively in humans, but influenza A has to mutate first.) For a bird flu subtype to become a true human virus—one that can be passed from person to person—it requires antigenic drift (slight genetic change) or antigenic shift, a more unusual process where bird and human viruses collide and merge.

Antigenic drift keeps scientists and vaccine makers on their toes, trying to match the yearly vaccine with the yearly antigenic variety of human flu. Theoretically, this merging or shifting of viral particles could happen in a person carrying a human flu who became infected simultaneously with a bird flu. However, most experts believe these shifts are much more common among pigs. Pigs make an excellent mixing bowl for influenza because they are susceptible to both bird and mammal varieties. A pig infected with both a human virus and a bird virus can develop a hybrid. But what sort of hybrid is very difficult to predict. Remember Vincent Price in *The Fly*? He went into a molecule mixer with an unnoticed fly and came out a monstrous killer with a fly's head and a human body. Meanwhile, somewhere out in the garden was a fly body with a human head that became the helpless victim of a spider. One message from this is that there is simply no controlling or predicting genetics. Similarly, if a hybrid flu bug manages to connect the deadly aspects of a bird flu with the "legs" of a human flu, it could become a monstrous human killer. However, this new subtype, being a mix of the two, could exhibit completely different qualities than the originals. A deadly bird flu could become a mild human flu, and a mild bird flu could become a deadly human one.

The novel H1N1 swine flu strain that caused the 2009 mild pandemic was likely formed in just this manner—a mixing of viral particles from swine, bird, and human influenza viruses.

A major human influenza A pandemic seems to occur, on average, three to four times each century. But no one can be certain when that pandemic will happen or which virus will be involved. Fortunately, the last three pandemics in the United States prior to the 2009 one had been getting progressively milder: from more than 500,000 dead in 1918 to around 70,000 in 1957–58 to between 25,000–50,000 in 1968–69. Was this a coincidence or was it the effects of modern medicine in combating the flu? The H1N1 swine flu pandemic would end up being even milder in the U.S. in terms of deaths, killing 12,500.

Slowing the rate of infection has more of an impact on reducing the death toll from a pandemic than on curing those who are infected. Fortunately for our collective survival, most viruses, as they mutate, become good at either spreading or killing, but not both. A virus that is easily and quickly spread tends not to be deadly. People who get only slightly sick are more likely to go about their daily life, spreading the disease everywhere they go. Rhinoviruses, which cause the common cold, are a good example. Almost everyone who comes in contact with the virus contracts it, but the symptoms are so mild that people decline to rest and instead go around spreading infection.

However, a virus that causes strong symptoms tends to be much slower in spreading. The symptoms themselves keep the patients at home. An example is the so called stomach virus (norovirus). Once a localized outbreak starts, usually from food handling, it quickly burns out, as most of those infected stay confined to their beds and bathrooms with nausea, vomiting, and diarrhea. While noroviruses are not deadly, and are actually quite common, the short period from exposure to severe symptoms is quick enough to slow its spread.

A pandemic needs to find just the right balance between the two. It must spread quickly, but also be deadly enough to claim a significant number of victims. Even the virus of 1918 killed only perhaps one in forty of those infected, but it made up for that by infecting hundreds of millions in a very short amount of time.

OTHER TWENTIETH CENTURY PANDEMICS

After the Spanish flu, the next global pandemic was much milder. The Asian flu was first identified in 1957. Thanks to the new virology of the time, this strain (H2N2) was identified immediately, and a vaccine went into production in May. Within a few months, a limited supply of vaccine became available.

As the infection spread through the fall, the rates of infection were highest among schoolchildren, young adults, and pregnant women, but the elderly had the highest rates of death. The pandemic peaked in midwinter. Close to 1 million people died globally, with 69,800 people dying in the United States—about double a normal flu year.

The most recent influenza pandemic before the current one came when the H3N2 strain appeared, first detected in Hong Kong in 1968 and now commonly referred to as the Hong Kong flu. It spread to the United States that fall, again peaking in winter, and again ultimately claiming its highest rate of victims among the elderly.

The Hong Kong flu continued the trend of weaker and weaker pandemics, with only 33,800 American deaths, and approximately 1 million deaths worldwide (still about double the number for the yearly flu outbreak). This pandemic was heading for its peak just as the holidays came, and may have been slowed as much by the closing of virus spreading classrooms as by the new technologies.

When a pandemic does occur, and an influenza A that we haven't seen before switches to humans, the bulk of the deaths has always been among those in developing countries. An underdeveloped public health system, lack of adequate medical care, and lack of effective means to spread knowledge and gain the cooperation of those at risk are the essential ingredients of a high death toll.

At the same time, looking at the history of influenza pandemics, there has been a positive trend. In industrialized nations, especially the United States, the interval between pandemics has been growing longer, the spread of the disease has been becoming slower, and the final mortality count has been getting smaller.

The coronavirus pandemic of 2020 would put an end to this trend in dramatic horrifying fashion.

THE H5N1 BIRD FLU

When an apparent new strain of avian flu appeared in Hong Kong in 1997, quick action was taken. Hong Kong's entire poultry population, about 1.5 million birds, was slaughtered, and many experts believed this aggressive culling prevented a wider pandemic. There was some concern at the time that eighteen humans had become infected with the virus and that six had died. Reassuring was the fact that each of these patients had become infected from direct contact with an infected bird, not an infected person.

Up to the end of 2003, H5N1 was considered a rare disease. But in mid December 2003 it reappeared in the Republic of Korea. By January 2004, Vietnam and Thailand both reported human cases of H5N1. In Japan it appeared in chickens, the first time that country had experienced a bird flu since 1925. In early 2004 it also turned up on a duck farm in China.

By May 2005, sporadic cases of people dying of bird flu had occurred in several Asian countries. By the end of August, the Philippines, the last Asian country without the disease, reported an outbreak in ducks and an unconfirmed case in a human. Russia, Tibet, and Kazakhstan also confirmed several cases in poultry. The virus seemed to be spreading from direct contact between wild, migratory waterfowl and domestic poultry. As fall approached, confirmed cases of the strain in birds had spread to Romania, Greece, and Turkey. Human cases were rare and sporadic, as they would continue to be for the next four years until the time of this writing. Aggressive culling (killing of birds) remained the first line of action in response to finding newly infected birds. Large commercial farmers were generally cooperative despite a loss of income. They understood the issue well and had trained workers to complete the culling. They used protective equipment and even Tamiflu for those workers who were most exposed.

Despite this, many Asian countries fighting the outbreak continued to have trouble controlling the spread of the disease in birds. This was because many of the owners of the birds were poor farmers who relied heavily on their small stock to survive. In several of the affected countries, as much as 80 percent of the total poultry production comes from small farms or even backyards.

The reluctance of small farmers to kill their entire flock also have translated into a reluctance to report potential infections. In addition, preventive measures were difficult for small farmers to undertake. In China alone, as many as 7 billion chickens are thought to be living on small farms in close proximity to humans, domestic animals, and perhaps most dangerously in terms of the potential for mutation, pigs. H5N1 mutated rapidly, but like all H5s had remained a massive killer of birds, not humans. That H5N1 has not evolved to spread easily from human to human was "no accident" according to Dr. Jeffrey Taubenberger of the National Institutes of Health. "The last several pandemics have all been H1, H2, H3," Taubenberger said to me in early 2006. "I am more concerned about another H1 mutating into a pandemic strain than I am about the H5N1 bird flu becoming the next pandemic." Taubenberger was right; this was exactly what happened. He was predicting the H1N1 swine flu pandemic we would be facing in 2009.

INFLUENZA A EVOLUTION IN HUMANS: 1918 VERSUS 1976

As I've discussed, the 1918 influenza virus, known as the Spanish flu or La Grippe, killed—by many estimates—more than 50 million people and was the most devastating pandemic in recorded history. During the outbreak, more people died of influenza in a single year than in the four years of the bubonic plague from 1347 to 1351. In the decades afterward, there were three main public reactions to influenza.

The first was denial. Before 2004, newspapers would stick any coverage they had about Asian bird flus deep in the unread pages of the international section. This reaction worried the public health community because there were thousands of flu bugs, and several mutated sufficiently to pass routinely from human to human and cause our yearly flu. The yearly flu, though not pandemic (involving multiple communities at once), was deadly enough to kill on average 34,000 people in the United States every year and hospitalize approximately 200,000.

The second reaction to the ghost of the 1918 killer flu was hysteria, or emotional forecasting based on no real information that this was going to be the year the Spanish flu—or worse—returned. The reincarnation in this case was first designated the H5N1 virus and then became the 2009

H1N1 swine flu; a real pandemic, but clearly nothing on the order of the 1918 scourge. In fact, the specter of the Spanish flu fueled many overreactions. The most prominent example occurred in 1976, when the swine flu made the jump from pigs to humans. This outbreak had many parallels with the 2005 excessive concern with the H5N1 bird flu; it never did wipe out millions as was feared, dead ending instead. The fear in 1976 was so great that more than 40 million people were vaccinated in a month in the United States using a hastily made vaccine that appears to have caused more than a thousand cases of Guillain Barré syndrome, a form of ascending paralysis from which some people never recover.

The third reaction to the ghost of 1918 was the most reasoned one, somewhere in the unexplored middle ground between denial and hysteria, and took into account both the fact that another pandemic was inevitable and that its magnitude and its timing were unknown.

This was why few anticipated the rapidity and ferocity of COVID-19.

In any case, in 2009, the plan of protection for a worst case scenario was woefully inadequate.

THE BLUE DEATH

In the fall of 1918, around the globe, perhaps beginning in the Indian Army, perhaps beginning in the U.S. Army, an infection took hold that was at first perceived to be no more than a cold. However, as it spread from America through Europe, it became more deadly. It quickly killed many who lived in the poor conditions of the combat trenches, but far more than that, it sped around the globe, killing tens of millions of people, including an estimated 17 million in India, where it did most of its damage.

Few countries were spared. Surprisingly, the flu was most deadly for young adults, between the ages of twenty and forty, rather than the very young and the elderly, whom most flus affect. Some experts have postulated in retrospect that it was the heightened immune response that healthy people can muster that somehow did them in. Their lungs may have filled up with infection fighting secretions they couldn't clear. Most experts agree that the most common cause of death was pneumonia and respiratory failure. Most likely, the pneumonia was a secondary bacterial pneumonia for which there were no antibiotic treatments available. The virus also appears to have caused neurological side effects in many survivors, including encephalopathy, an inflammation of the brain that often leads to permanent disabilities.

In the end, the Spanish flu infected at least 28 percent of all Americans, and at least 500,000 died. Half of the American soldiers who died in Europe died from influenza rather than from combat.

As noted in the Journal of the American Medical Association's final edition of 1918, "1918 has gone: a year momentous as the termination of the most cruel war in the annals of the human race; a year which marked, the end at least for a time, of man's destruction of man; unfortunately a year in which developed a most fatal infectious disease causing the death of hundreds of thousands of human beings. Medical science for four and one half years devoted itself to putting men on the firing line and keeping them there. Now it must turn with its whole might to combating the greatest enemy of all: infectious disease."

Even with the Spanish flu, by some estimates the worst of all plagues, most victims recovered, and their experience generally was a more intense version of the expected week long course of fever, aches, chills, and nausea that characterized all influenza. But a substantial minority endured much worse. They were exhausted, with earaches, headaches, high fever, and difficult breathing.

Doctors with little experience diagnosing viruses (they still didn't really know what a virus was) often confused the Spanish flu with a cold until the patients were very sick.

Some patients died rapidly, sometimes overnight. They reportedly turned cyanotic (meaning they turned blue), struggled for air, and were choked by their blood tinged secretions. As the disease progressed and pneumonia set in, they sometimes began to bleed profusely—from the nose, the ears, and the mouth. Some still recovered, but when cyanosis appeared, physicians treated patients as terminal. Autopsies show a disease that ravaged almost every internal organ.

The pandemic circled the globe, often following trade routes and shipping lines. Outbreaks coursed through North America, Europe, Asia, Brazil, and the South Pacific. Soldiers spread it to faraway lands on ships. The Committee on Atmosphere and Man concluded in 1923 that humidity was a factor in the spread of the disease.

As I discussed in chapter 1, the origin of the Spanish flu is not known, although the current prevailing theory is that it started in China. In the spring of 1918 it first arrived in the United States in Kansas and in U.S. military camps, where it wasn't acknowledged initially, the focus instead being on winding down the war.

The war brought a second wave of the virus back in September, and by then it appeared much more deadly, perhaps because of further mutations to the viral structure. It first arrived in Boston in late August, and by October two hundred thousand in the United States were dead. The U.S. Public Health Service (USPHS) was in charge of coordinating care among the states, but the wartime shortage of doctors, and especially nurses, made this care very difficult to deliver on a consistent basis. Congress appropriated $1 million to the USPHS, but didn't appropriate funds specifically for influenza research. The USPHS did appoint a director for influenza in each state but wasn't effective in coordinating care. People often died of dehydration, starvation, and poor care, rather than the flu itself. Disorganization and lack of solid disseminated information contributed to the problem. Doctors, with no vaccines or treatments available and a poor understanding of the disease, turned desperate, even using unproven nonviral based vaccines (often targeting some imagined bacteria). This was at a time when most doctors were still taught that bleeding a patient was the best cure for pneumonia. Doctors urged cities to quarantine the sick and restrict attendance at public gatherings, but wartime rallies and draft registrations supervened.

Urban conditions were crowded, poorly ventilated, and filthy—conducive to the spread of disease. Schools, cinemas, churches, and public meetinghouses were supposed to be closed, and attempts were made to force infected patients into hospital wards, but many of these ordinances were ignored by people who didn't realize the danger they were in. Many cities refused to shut their public transit systems until hundreds of sick transit workers forced them to do so. Boston ignored the epidemic initially, because of the city's seeming good health, and the country only began to pay attention in late September, when the disease had already spread as far as Seattle.

Medical personnel discovered that having infected people wear surgical masks, helped limit the spread of infection—until they ran out of gauze to make the masks. They understood that administering oxygen to patients in distress was helpful, but they didn't have the means to administer it to even a small percentage of those who needed it.

The Red Cross responded to the nursing shortage by asking for volunteers and by creating the National Committee on Influenza. Emergency hospitals were created to take in those sick with influenza as well as those arriving sick from overseas. With one quarter of the United States and one fifth of the world infected, it was impossible to escape it, though the wealthy and the famous were fairly successful at sequestering themselves. But even President Woodrow Wilson caught influenza in early 1919 while negotiating the Treaty of Versailles.

Scientists, having recently accepted germ theory, worked unsuccessfully on a vaccine. Public health officials, capitalizing on restrictions already in place for the war, tried to restrict movement between U.S. cities. Railroads wouldn't accept passengers without signed documentation attesting to no infection. But overall, the public health response was characterized by confusion, disorganization, ineffectiveness, and edicts that weren't followed.

And then, as quickly as it had come, perhaps aided by the coming of spring, when flu viruses traditionally fail to thrive, the Spanish flu died out. Later research—much of it conducted by Dr. Jeffrey Taubenberger at the Air Force Institute of Pathology over the past two decades—identified the virus that caused the Spanish flu. He also described the bacteria like pneumonia that caused its secondary, life-threatening complications.

Public health officials are far better off in 2020 than in 1918 at emphasizing public education and promoting public cooperation. One can only speculate about what would have happened in 1918 if doctors had available even a tenth of the technology and methods we have today.

At the same time, the world is much more densely populated, and air travel allows people to journey (and potentially spread disease) to far off places in only hours. But while a plane covers a lot of distance very quickly, a 1918 military ship in the middle of the high seas, densely packed with exhausted young men eating and sleeping in close quarters, made for a better environment to grow and spread a virus.

1976 SWINE FLU

On February 5, 1976, nineteen year old Private David Lewis of Massachusetts told his drill instructor at Fort Dix that he felt tired and weak. Nevertheless, he participated in a training hike, and within twenty four hours he was dead. I spoke with several sources in the military who said that the initial reaction on the part of the military was simple caution, as laboratory tests were run. But fears soon exploded. Two weeks after Lewis's death, health officials from the Centers for Disease Control and Prevention (CDC), calling Lewis's the "index case" and having isolated five hundred other cases of what they called "swine flu" in other recruits who hadn't gotten sick (serological testing showed exposure) and four who had, disclosed to the American public that there was concern about a possible epidemic. Press conferences and public panic ensued as health officials reasoned that any flu that was able to reach so many people so fast was capable of becoming a worldwide plague.

With the specter of 1918 firmly in their minds, public health officials quickly considered the possibility of mass inoculations before the next flu season, worrying that as in 1918 (as well as 1957 and 1968), the flu virus might get stronger by its second season, or wave.

Some experts maintained that this was a great example of America's public health community acting in advance of what could easily have been a new plague. At the time, the Spanish flu was wrongly understood to have developed from exposure to pigs, as the 1976 swine flu strain clearly had. The accepted theory in 1976 was that bird flus and human flus commingle in pigs and that the required mutation necessary to give a bird flu "human legs" occurs most easily by that exchange of genetic material in a pig's blood (antigenic shift). This theory is still believed to be a likely method of transmitting many animal flu viruses to humans. In fact, frequent exposure to swine flu viruses leads to seroconversion (making antibodies) in food handlers and pig farmers.

Back in 1976, operating on the assumption that the swine flu virus that had been discovered was very similar to the 1918 flu bug, public health officials and leaders, and subsequently the public, were all worried. No one knew how the swine flu had gotten to Fort Dix, but health officials were concerned that it could spread rapidly from there.

Weeks after Private Lewis died, doctors from the CDC, including the director, Dr. David Spencer; the sagacious polio vaccine inventors Jonas Salk and Albert Sabin; and other officials met in Washington, D.C., to decide what to do. While they were concerned about swine flu, they also were concerned that attempts to rapidly immunize the public against it would interrupt work on many other diseases. And while they could only imagine the complaints doctors would face if an epidemic broke out and vaccines weren't ready, they couldn't help wonder what would happen if everyone was inoculated for a plague that didn't happen.

By March 1976, Dr. Spencer had lined up most of the medical establishment behind his plan to ask the president for $135 million to mass-vaccinate the country.

But there may have been more to it than simple medical concerns. In Pure Politics and Impure Science, Arthur M. Silverstein suggests that presidential politics played a heavy role in this decision, as President Gerald Ford, up for reelection and under the influence of America's big drug manufacturers, wanted to be seen as a hero.

On March 24, the day after a surprise loss to Ronald Reagan in the North Carolina Republican primary, Ford made his announcement to the public and prepared to take this battle to Congress. Meanwhile, the drug makers were insisting that the government take liability for any harmful side effects from a hastily made vaccine. Congressional hearings stretched on into the early summer, with some "doubting Thomases" pointing out that swine flu hadn't extended beyond Fort Dix in its "first wave."

Ultimately, the president and his experts prevailed, and on August 12, Congress approved the funding. Dr. W. Delano Meriwether of the Department of Health, Education, and Welfare, a thirty-three-year old physician and world-class sprinter, was put in charge of the project and given until the end of the year to inoculate all 220 million Americans against swine flu.

When insurance companies refused to provide coverage to the vaccine manufacturers, the government finally agreed to accept liability for claims of adverse events. This obstacle having been cleared, the National Influenza Immunization Program (NIIP) officially started in October 1976.

By October 1 the serum was ready, and the public health system had organized doctors, nurses, and paraprofessionals to administer the shots. Within days, several people who had received the shot fell seriously ill. Three elderly people in Pennsylvania had their shots and died a few hours later of heart attacks, causing the program to be immediately suspended in that state.

Other states pressed on, even as more reports of adverse side effects came out. The number of vaccinations given each week increased rapidly from less than 1 million in early October to more than 4 million in the later weeks of the month, reaching a peak of more than 6 million doses a week by the middle of November 1976. The NIIP was unique in the annals of epidemiology: an organized surveillance effort was in place from the very beginning, and more than 40 million people were vaccinated during the short time the NIIP was in effect. However, on December 16, 1976, the NIIP was suspended following reports from more than ten states of Guillain Barré syndrome (GBS) in vaccinees. By January 1977, more than five hundred cases of GBS had been reported, with twenty five deaths. The government suspended the program. Millions of dollars in lawsuits followed.

THE SWINE FLU NEVER CAME

In 1976, our public health officials pulled off an astonishing public health feat to counter what they thought was an emerging plague based on 1918 fears. But rather than learn from this event today, we leave it buried in history. Public health officials both then and now speak with an apparent certainty that does not always reflect the amount of speculation involved. Our reaction to the 1976 swine flu showed not only you can rush to judgment, wasting time and money ramping up for a worst case scenario that never comes, but that in doing so, there may be significant costs to people's health.

The swine flu scare helped foster cynicism and distrust of federal policy makers and health officials. But Joseph Califano, who subsequently became secretary of the Department of Health, Education, and Welfare under President Carter, continued to maintain that doctors had had no choice but to err on the side of caution, and should do so again if faced with the threat of another killer plague with the potential to kill millions.

GUILLAIN-BARRÉ SYNDROME

Guillain Barré syndrome (GBS) is a fairly uncommon neurologic disorder characterized by sudden muscular weakness, especially in the hands and feet, though in more severe cases the muscles of breathing are involved. Symptoms of ascending paralysis may progress for up to ten days. Patients often improve, and recovery tends to occur within three months. Some unusual cases have been difficult to diagnose. The exact cause of GBS remains unknown. It was always believed to be due to a virus, but more recently it has been seen as an immunological reaction to an invading agent (including virus particles).

For the first time ever, a nationwide surveillance system was established to evaluate illnesses that might be due to the vaccination program.

The network was coordinated by the CDC, with state and local participation mandatory. A registration consent form had to be signed by all vaccinees. Any illness serious enough to cause hospitalization had to be telephoned in to the CDC.

In August 1977 the results were released to the public. In 1979 Alexander Langmuir, director of the epidemiology branch of the National Communicable Disease Center in Atlanta, presented a preliminary report. Based on the weekly numbers of vaccinations, a comparison of observed with expected cases showed that the relative risk of acquiring GBS during the six weeks after vaccination was about ten times the expectation. Langmuir concluded that the vaccine contained a "trigger element" leading to GBS in 1 in 100,000 of those who received the vaccine. Also in 1979, Dr. Lawrence Schonberger and his collaborators at the CDC presented an additional analysis of the national surveillance data of cases. A total of 1,098 cases of GBS had been reported to the CDC during the four months under investigation. (No doubt many more cases were not reported.) Subsequently, lawsuits led to reevaluation of the cases by a government panel formed by Langmuir. The apparent association between the vaccine and the development of GBS was again confirmed.

Soon after the publication of this study, Nathan Mantel, at the time a professor of statistics at George Washington University, released criticisms suggesting that the number of cases that occurred late had been underreported by both Langmuir and Schonberger and that more compensation should have been considered. However, subsequent studies, in Michigan and Ohio in 1984, confirmed that the main risk period had really been six weeks after vaccination, as had been reported.

In a key finding, both Schonberger and Langmuir had discovered that among cases of GBS, those in the vaccinated group had a much lower incidence of another explanation for it, namely an acute viral type illness. The "trigger element" in 1976 could have been one of the proteins from the virus used to make the vaccine. Antibodies against peripheral nerves were produced as a result, causing the ascending paralysis that patients experienced. Subsequent flu vaccines have not shown an increased incidence of GBS (except for a possible slight increase in 1992 and 1993).

A Harvard study in 1997 by Elissa Laitin and Elise Pelletier reviewed all the prior studies and concluded that there was strong evidence to show a causal link between the swine flu vaccine and GBS. This conclusion was possible thanks to the well organized surveillance effort in 1976, a key tool of epidemiology.

At the same time, many cases probably went unrecognized or unreported at the time. As an example, I received this recent correspondence: "I was stationed at Fort Dix in early 1976 as a fresh young recruit during the swine flu period. We were vaccinated with a vaccine. I become very ill during this period and was hospitalized at the main base hospital. Please, I was hoping you could provide me with the name of the condition or disease which causes a type of paralysis."

One positive outcome of the swine flu vaccine/GBS disaster was the development of the National Vaccine Injury Compensation Program in 1988, which compensates people for vaccine related injuries or death.

The swine flu lesson is about cost and benefit. The ghosts of 1918 teach valuable lessons, but these ghosts can both help provoke a hasty reaction to a new virus—as well as warn us for a worst case scenario such as COVID-19.

Careful consideration should always be given to the science on all sides. In the case of swine flu in 1976, there simply wasn't enough scientific evidence to back the conviction many officials had that a giant pandemic was imminent. No one wanted to admit that they were speculating about the 1918 virus and applying that scenario to the 1976 swine flu, a trend that we seem poised to repeat.

2009

Speculation is not science. And science is an ongoing series of observations, not an assertion that is blindly adhered to ("The world is flat") despite corrective facts. In 1976, such a course correction should have been made when the supposed "first wave" of the outbreak that was to approximate the one of 1918 never made it out of Fort Dix. Ignoring that important fact showed strong conviction, but it wasn't good science.

In 2009, when we again faced an inflamed situation, with plans afoot to ramp up vaccine production against a virus that was spreading widely but was not very deadly—perhaps the mildest of pandemics—we had to incorporate the lessons of 1976 as well as those of 1918. The lessons of 1918 were best learned when contrasted with the massive fear driven reaction in 1976.

A major problem back in 1918 was that the country wasn't focused on public health and instead continued to rely on old solutions that didn't work. By contrast, the world in 2009 was much more overcrowded and easily traveled but also has the antibiotics, steroids, heart and diabetes medication, sanitation, and public health that 1918 lacked. Despite these essential differences, nevertheless we invoked 1918 and instantly reacted to whatever threat we thought we faced.

There are the long term preparedness issues that won't go away. These involve improving hospital and emergency responder readiness as well as upgrading how we make vaccine through the use of our latest technologies.

SWINE FLU–
THE LAST PANDEMIC

APRIL 2009: THE WORRIED BUS DRIVER

My son's school bus driver had told me several months earlier that he was having problems sleeping at night. I had offered advice on developing a sleep ritual, and he soon began looking more relaxed. But when the swine flu scare first hit in late April, he was again appearing fatigued. He said he was worried about the risks that going to school might pose to students. I was worried too, not about swine flu, but about his driving my son and other children in his sleepless condition.

I told him that the flu appeared to be mild and that there were only a few cases in the city. The danger was minimal, I said. He didn't seem reassured—and he wasn't the only one. As the new virus continued to spread, I was having difficulty helping my patients, friends, and relatives put the fear of this new flu strain in perspective.

With previous scares, such as those connected to bird flu, anthrax contamination, mad cow disease, and the West Nile virus, I'd been able to point out that the pathogen wasn't spreading person to person and was therefore of limited concern. But this wasn't the case with the new H1N1 flu.

I tried my best to explain the science of flu to the bus driver as well as to my patients. A flu virus is a package of genetic material (called RNA) inside an envelope. "H" refers to hemagglutinin, the protein on the envelope that enables the flu to attach to your cell and inject itself inside. The

"N" is neuraminidase, the protein that helps a flu virus break off from your cell and move on to a new cell. The new strain appeared to be the result of what is known as a "triple-reassortant" swine influenza strain (with mixed genes from human, swine, and bird flu viruses) that had been confined mainly to pigs (pigs are a mixing vessel for flu) until it combined again, with a Eurasian swine flu strain. This new strain—though still mild in severity—began passing easily from human to human, causing the March 2009 outbreak in Mexico and the United States.

I also explained to my patients that though this virus was transmitted fairly easily, like many influenzas it appeared to lack certain proteins that made other flu viruses more deadly. One of these, known as PB1 2, weakens the immune system by attacking the protective covering of cell mitochondria (motors). All the pandemic flus of the twentieth century made this enzyme, but the new swine flu strain did not, which was good news. Another enzyme the virus lacked (luckily) is responsible for blocking the body's production of interferon, a crucial chemical that helps us keep the flu virus from spreading easily from cell to cell.

An article in the New England Journal of Medicine suggested that many people (those born prior to 1957) might have a partial immunity to this strain because of prior exposure to other related H1 viruses that were circulating at the time. This theory seemed plausible as the new strain spread and the elderly were the least affected. The new virus also seemed to be following a Darwinian principle of survival of the fittest. Fitness, though it helps a virus to spread, doesn't imply lethality; in fact, it often implies the opposite. (Viruses that kill their hosts can't easily jump to another host.) But flu viruses mutate often, and I couldn't reassure the bus driver or anyone else with absolute certainty that this weak influenza wouldn't return in a more ferocious form in the fall.

This uncertainty scared people. To make it worse, grainy photos of stricken patients during the 1918 Spanish flu pandemic were often shown on TV when health officials and some media outlets trumped up the latest influenza concern. The comparisons weren't fair on many levels. Back in 1918 we didn't have antibiotics, antivirals, or treatments for heart disease or asthma. The majority of those who died likely succumbed to bacterial pneumonia. Death certificates for the Spanish flu listed pneumonia as the cause in the majority of cases.

Influenza weakens you. It is generally not influenza, but an accompanying condition, that hospitalizes or kills a victim. We have a variety of treatments for these conditions that we lacked back in 1918. But the public worried about what it couldn't see—about what apparently came from a loud, smelly creature such as a pig. It worried about a contagion that initially appeared to come from a foreign country. Even the word "pandemic" (from the Greek meaning "everyone") scared people, especially as the World Health Organization (WHO) didn't describe it well in terms of either number of cases or deaths; it was just a ubiquitous term floating over us.

The new swine flu strain—with fewer than 10,000 confirmed cases by the beginning of May 2009—was already on the verge of being labeled a full scale pandemic by WHO criteria. It was hard to conceive of where the bubonic plague, which killed 75 million in the fourteenth century, would fit on such a scale. People quickly developed the false sense that the virus was everywhere.

And then, just as quickly, the obsessive worry left us. The message got out through the media in mid May that this was a virus to monitor and be prepared for, but not to panic over. Unless there were bodies on stretchers, the low news ratings wouldn't sustain continued coverage.

As we bounced from one health scare to the next, it didn't seem that we were learning anything. My son's bus driver was relieved by the media drop off, and he was sleeping better at night—until the day when he wasn't. "My ribs are hurting me," he explained. "My doctor is concerned about my pancreas. I can't sleep on my side." I looked at him. He imagined dangers that weren't there. But he also had real health problems. His pancreas was something that perhaps should cause him to worry.

By mid May 2009, sniffles cases were no longer filling our emergency rooms and getting in the way of sicker patients. At the height of the early flu scare, a patient of mine had arrived in the emergency room with several broken bones, a head injury, and profuse bleeding, yet was back burnered in favor of "flu sufferers" who later tested negative. She waited for more than an hour, experiencing further bleeding and risking infection from her open wounds. She was ultimately okay, but the delay was dangerous. Although tracking the new flu was certainly in the interest of public health, the symptoms being reported by sniffling worriers didn't warrant this kind of emergency room triage. Luckily, by mid May this massive overreaction was completely over—at least for the time being.

THE WHO AND THE FLU

The World Health Organization's FluNet, a contagion control network, not only helps to track influenza but also provides essential knowledge of prevailing strains to help manufacturers prepare the yearly vaccine. And the WHO's quick boots on the ground response to flu was instrumental in following and analyzing the initial A(H1N1) swine flu outbreak. But the WHO also was engaged in the kind of scary speculation that was unscientific and fueled the initial panic.

As the number of confirmed swine flu cases in the world reached close to 10,000 by the middle of May 2009, WHO flu chief Keiji Fukuda was already busy speculating wildly at a press conference on May 7 that this outbreak could end up infecting up to 2 billion people—a third of the world's population. He said he based this prediction on the behavior of previous pandemics, but the 1968 Hong Kong flu, the last true pandemic, infected far fewer than that.

It was far too early to be speculating on the extent of spread or potential deadliness. Further, it was likely that the death rate was actually much lower than had been reported, because the vast majority of mild cases had not been confirmed and would not be confirmed. Flu outbreaks tended to wane in the summer months, as respiratory viruses were transmitted more easily during periods of cold weather or low humidity. But pandemic strains tended to persist and to make an appearance at summer camps. Since this was a new strain with pandemic potential even though it was mild, many scientists did expect it to continue to infect people through June and July in the United States. This concern turned out to be well founded.

It was wise to be tracking this virus into the Southern Hemisphere as that region's winter and flu season started, and it was wise to be preparing a vaccine. But the WHO's tendency to make sweeping, unsubstantiated predictions was not particularly helpful, and it never had been. Back in the fall of 2005, David Nabarro, the United Nations' systems coordinator for avian and human influenza, had predicted that 5 million to 150 million could die of H5N1 bird flu. In the spring of 2003, the WHO, predicting a 5 percent to 6 percent death rate from severe acute respiratory syndrome (SARS) and concerned about a massive pandemic, had issued its first travel advisory and enacted a global surveillance network. This effort cost the world's economies more than $30 billion. In the end, SARS infected only 8,400 people, killing 774 worldwide, before the WHO finally concluded that this virus didn't spread easily through the air.

Part of the problem existed with the Epidemic and Pandemic Alert and Response system WHO used to warn us about pandemics, focusing attention on and then ultimately asking for billions of dollars in funding. The WHO's global influenza preparedness plan was updated in 2005 in response to the H5N1 avian flu scare. But in part because it was a response to a scare rather than a real pandemic with documented cases, it lacked any quantification of either the extent of spread or the severity of the virus. The 2009 swine flu outbreak, the first time the revised flu alert system had been used, revealed that the system suffered from ineffectiveness due to its vagueness and premature trigger. This was why we found ourselves in May 2009 on the verge of declaring a pandemic for swine flu so quickly. Phase 5 (out of a possible 6) of the WHO pandemic alert for the flu virus states, "human-to-human spread of the virus into at least two countries in one WHO region . . . while most countries will not be affected at this stage, the declaration of Phase 5 is a strong signal that a pandemic is imminent."

"Imminent" was another term that had the potential to alarm us. But the biggest problem of all was the premature worldwide alert for a problem that was not yet that extensive and that didn't appear deadly. If this was how the WHO geared up in advance of a real problem, how could it possibly retain the resources to deal with the world's real ongoing pandemics, such as HIV/AIDS, malaria, tuberculosis, diarrheal diseases, or malnutrition? Or for that matter, how would it react to a real massive pandemic like coronavirus in 2020? I will explore that in Part two.

A total of 33 million people were suffering from HIV in the world, with more than 3 million deaths per year. There were 300 million to 500 million cases of malaria per year according to the WHO, with 1.5 million to 2.7 million deaths. More than a third of the world was starving, and the WHO reported that at least 15 million children die of hunger each year.

Did we want precious WHO resources so easily diverted from these children to a postmodern panic born of our obsession with a new 2009 flu strain?

THE CDC

I was more affected by President Obama's statement in response to the emerging swine flu threat that we should all wash our hands, than I was to Vice President Biden's famous misstatement about not flying on planes for fear of flu.

Let me explain. Clearly, the president was correct; we carry many bacteria and viruses on our hands, and in fact most of our stomach viruses as well as cold viruses are passed back and forth this way. It was hard to fault anyone for recommending hand-washing—in fact, it was a good thing—but consider that Obama's statement carried the subliminal message that we might all be carrying this virus, despite the fact that in May 2009 the statistical chances of that remained extremely low.

The president followed that up by asking Congress for $1.5 billion to prepare us for this flu, an amount that seemed totally reasonable.

But stockpiles of the antiflu drug Tamiflu would have to be discarded if they weren't used in five years, and this was a distinct possibility. We had no idea what the extent of spread or severity of this swine flu virus would be. Preparing a vaccine seemed especially wise, but taking needed resources away from current pandemics such as TB, HIV, or even the yearly flu did not.

The Centers for Disease Control and Prevention was front and center during the initial stages of the swine flu outbreak, and they were very effective at identifying and tracking the virus, but like the WHO, the CDC was less effective at explaining it in context during press conferences (media outlets picked up the conferences, and the message was instantly amplified).

The CDC was getting a new director, New York City health commissioner Thomas Frieden, a smart epidemiologist who ended up proving to be as effective behind a microphone as he was in the field.

SWINE FLU IN PERSPECTIVE

At the beginning of the outbreak, when the number of documented U.S. cases of the new flu strain had still been fewer than five hundred and the WHO had first considered raising its pandemic alert to the highest level, pork manufacturers had complained that the name "swine flu" was misleading. Though the virus may have originated in pigs, pork was not the problem, they said. The virus spread from Mexico to the United States, Europe, and New Zealand by human to-human transmission.

Pork to human transmission was just one of many misperceptions that had developed once the flu strain was discovered. As I have discussed, parallels were too quickly drawn between this emerging virus and the 1918 Spanish flu. But the 1918 virus was an exotic, birdlike virus that made the jump to humans. The theory—later disproved—that it was actually a swine flu virus had been part of what had triggered the swine flu panic in 1976.

The new flu strain was clearly more virulent and transmissible than the 1976 strain. But it had seemed to be more deadly when it first emerged in Mexico. As it adapted to human to-human transmission, it was likely becoming less powerful.

The CDC announced that the virus appeared to have a 25 percent attack rate, similar to the yearly flu, meaning that for every person who had it, one out of four of their contacts would get it. But the misperception initially was that the new flu was far more contagious than that.

What we needed as the number of swine flu cases rose through the late spring of 2009 was to keep things in perspective. Even as the number of unconfirmed cases passed 1 million, the number of people who had died from this virus was still fewer than three hundred.

ON SWINE FLU AND TAMIFLU

Back in late April, during the heart of the early swine flu scare, I had brought some samples of the antiviral drug Tamiflu (oseltamivir) to a TV studio to use as a prop on a show. But when I went to leave the show, I discovered that one of the producers had rifled through the box, and most of the samples were gone. This piracy was due to the fear of flu.

As I've mentioned, influenza has two main proteins on its surface envelope. One of them, neuraminidase (N), allows the virus to break off and move on to the next cell. The antiviral drugs Tamiflu and Relenza (zanamivir) are neuraminidase inhibitors, meaning that they stop this enzyme from working so the flu virus can't detach and move on successfully.

These drugs had the potential to help slow the progress of the new outbreak and potentially save lives, especially in advance of a vaccine. It was important for governments to stockpile the antiflu drugs, but it was equally as important that individuals didn't hoard them or use them prematurely. Overuse could lead to drug resistance, and then the drugs wouldn't be useful if the outbreak continued to spread.

CLOSE THE SCHOOLS

My sister teaches college in California, and throughout May 2009 she was forwarding me e mail announcements about influenza A(H1N1) appearing in her school, yet the school remained open. I was soon experiencing the same kind of delay here in New York City, where the Department of Health, still led by newly appointed CDC director Thomas Frieden, worked together with the Department of Education to close more than twenty schools with either documented H1N1 swine flu or increased amounts of influenza like illness. Yet the vast majority of schools stayed open.

In just three weeks we had gone from a vast overreaction to a the coast is clear underreaction. This is a penalty for panic. When public health grabbed the media spotlight and started press-conferencing, it soon lost the opportunity to properly inform. If only this mild virus hadn't been so mischaracterized as deadly and omnipresent from the start, we might have become less openly dismissive of it when we saw that the bodies weren't piling up.

Humans have a limited attention span, and our fear radar is soon diverted elsewhere. By the time fear might even be appropriate to protect us from a risk, we have already turned away. In late May the New York City Health Department began to receive justified criticism from parents for being too slow to close the schools and for being inconsistent in their policies. Mrs. Bonnie Wiener (her husband, Mitchell, an assistant principal in Queens contracted A(H1N1) and died in May 2009) insisted that schools should have been closed sooner. Schools are places where infections can thrive.

I spoke to one parent of a ten year old who has stayed home from New York City's P.S. 175 with a documented case of influenza A, yet the school remained open, and the father, who lacked insurance, was unable to get Tamiflu from city hospitals for either his child or himself.

This was wrong. The indecision and delay by health and education officials in closing schools risked breeding a new wave of fear among parents. Frieden and his troops were too slow. Schools needed to consider closing in advance of the flu horses getting out of the barn, especially when there was no vaccine available to help provide a herd immunity to those who might be exposed. The close contact and shared surfaces at schools made them petri dishes for spreading flu. In contrast to the public schools was the shining example of the Horace Mann School in Riverdale, New York, where the school closed for flu related illness on May 20, 2009, in advance of any confirmed cases. The headmaster, Dr. Tom Kelly, used the occasion as a learning experience for the entire school. "In the end, swine flu or not, we're going to emerge a healthier school with better health related practices," Kelly said.

The school was vacated for a week and disinfected. Learning continued online, as Kelly and the department heads created an interactive center to provide information about influenza. By the time one young student was hospitalized with likely H1N1, the other students were out of harm's way.

Kelly's wise, courageous decision no doubt helped others outside the school, those with chronic illnesses who might have come in contact with flu ridden students if the school had stayed open. No matter how mild this flu was in its first wave, it was still a risk to those with weakened immune systems. Kelly's move was a reminder that we are all part of one large community where responsibility implies sober risk assessment without either frantic overreaction or the underreaction of denial.

He developed an even more extensive plan for the COVID pandemic of 2020, as I will discuss in Part Two.

JUNE 2009: THE FIRST WAVE?

As schools began to let out for the summer, H1N1 continued to infect people. The CDC estimated that the total number of cases in the United States alone was approaching 1 million. The disease continued to be quite mild, with fifteen deaths in the United States, but it was looking like it would continue into the summer, as the flu pandemic of 1957 had done. Generally in the summer flu viruses don't do as well because (1) they survive longer in cooler, drier air and (2) schools—incubators for the spread of flu—let out, but in the case of a novel virus with no vaccine and little or no immunity, an epidemic could continue through the summer and then combust in the fall. In 1957 there were summer outbreaks, which included church gatherings, international students in Iowa, and schoolchildren in Louisiana. In 1957, the pandemic really took hold in

September, which is several months earlier than the peak of the typical yearly flu.

Pandemic flus usually start much earlier than the yearly flu, and generally hospitalize and kill younger patients, probably because these are the patients who most lack immunity due to lack of exposure to previous related flu viruses. The yearly flu kills 34,000 in the United States and more than 500,000 people worldwide, but more than 90 percent of these deaths are of the elderly and provoked by associated conditions such as bacterial pneumonia. The 1957 pandemic caused nearly 70,000 U.S. deaths, and a large number was not of the elderly.

Pandemics tend to come in waves. Lone Simonsen, longtime flu epidemiologist at the National Institutes of Health (NIH) and currently a professor at George Washington University, has studied this phenomenon. She wrote about it in the New England Journal of Medicine in May 2009 and discussed her findings with me in an interview. In 1918, a milder wave of flu cases famously occurred in early spring, followed by the deadly surge in the fall and winter that killed more than 50 million people worldwide. In 1957, Asian flu was mild in China, before the summer outbreaks in the United States followed by the more severe flu season. The 1957 pandemic was recurrent, with three waves over five years, returning in 1959 and 1962. The 1968 Hong Kong flu pandemic, the mildest of the century, had two waves in Great Britain, with 85 percent of the deaths occurring in the winter of 1969.

On June 11, the 2009 A (H1N1) flu finally qualified as a pandemic in the eyes of the WHO. Though there were still fewer than two hundred related deaths in the world by this time, the fact that it was spreading easily in two regions of the world met the definition of a WHO pandemic.

By early July there still were only 429 deaths globally, though the virus had most likely spread to more than 1 million people in the United States alone.

Gearing up for the fall season, the U.S. Congress allocated $1 billion for vaccine ingredients, and Department of Health and Human Services secretary Katherine Sebelius, echoing President Obama's sentiment, indicated that $7.5 billion more would be allocated for emergency preparedness. A national vaccination program was envisioned, with 600 million doses of a two shot vaccine to be produced by sometime in the fall. Several manufacturers were involved, including Novartis AG, which had produced its first batch using cell culture technology (where the vaccine is grown in mammalian cells rather than the laborious, outdated hen culture medium that most vaccine manufacturers still used). Other vaccine manufactures, including Sanofi Pasteur, GSK, and Baxter, were using the traditional method. Protein Sciences Corp. was producing vaccine at a rapid pace (100,000 doses per week) using more modern genetic techniques. By July 2009, twenty-four controlled trials were ongoing in humans, and by the end of the month nine were completed. The vaccine appeared to be very well tolerated. It remained to be seen whether one or two doses were going to be necessary to achieve immunity.

JULY 2009

For three summers, my twelve year old son Joshua had attended Camp Modin, a beautiful camp in rural Maine. This year, when we dropped him off at the northbound bus, something was different: the counselors were taking children's temperatures before letting them on board. It seemed a wise precaution, as the new influenza A(H1N1) swine flu strain continues to spread and the weather in Maine in June was cool this year, which could facilitate an outbreak of the virus. But as a physician who has studied the flu for many years, I was still worried. An infected person can be contagious even if he doesn't have a fever.

My concern was justified. Three days after camp started, I called the camp director, Howard Salzberg, and discovered that he was beside himself. One of the parents, another physician, had used Tylenol to deliberately suppress his child's fever so he wouldn't be held back. There were already sixteen cases of the flu, confirmed by the Maine Center for Disease Control and Prevention to be the H1N1 swine flu strain. Desperate to contain the infection, and at the advice of the CDC, Howard had created a quarantine bunk for the sick and was having all the bunks cleaned with hospital grade disinfectant. One other tool could help stem the spread of infection—but using it would go against CDC protocol.

The CDC has a national policy to reserve the antiflu drug Tamiflu— which works by blocking the enzyme (neuraminidase) that allows the flu virus to detach from one human cell and spread to the next one—for only severe cases. But with the new pandemic strain circling the globe and more than 1 million people already likely infected in the United States by July, it seemed to me that it was time for our public health authorities to employ a more aggressive strategy. Clinical trials had shown that Tamiflu, when taken within forty-eight hours of exposure, is 92 percent effective at preventing flu in adults and 82 percent effective in children. Since we didn't yet have a vaccine, I felt that the best strategy was to use the drug, which decreases the severity and the duration of the illness and helps prevent people who are in contact with flu patients from getting sick themselves. I e mailed the camp parents to let them know that Tamiflu is well tolerated and safe and that I was starting my son Josh on a ten day course of it; it would be wise, I recommended, for them to do the same. If Josh came home with the flu, I reasoned, he would put his four year old brother Sam, who had asthma, at risk for a more serious case. I believed my situation was not unique, and prescriptions were soon flooding the camp's fax machine; of the 380 campers, 250 were started on the drug, as were more than 100 staffers.

I also sent my son Josh a separate e mail telling him that unless the Tamiflu worked to control the outbreak, I was coming to Maine to bring him home. I suggested he have his counselor contact me if he wanted to come home. My son, a tough, clearheaded child who didn't give in to fear or emotion, did not have his counselor contact me.

At the same time that the prescriptions were pouring in, the Maine CDC asked to speak to me, since this was not its usual protocol. It was holding Tamiflu in reserve for the sickest cases. But our children had no immunity to this new strain of flu. Though most of the stricken Modin campers were only mildly ill, how did we know when it would reach a child with a chronic illness such as asthma that might not yet be diagnosed? Since campers could have had those conditions but not yet have been diagnosed for them, it made a lot of sense to use Tamiflu to reduce the amount of circulating virus and dramatically reduce the risk of hospitalization or death. I also had explained to the director of the camp that most of the studies using antivirals as a preventive, conducted in nursing homes, were likely applicable to the camp environment, since kids were crammed in bunks, just as patients in nursing homes live close together.

As someone who has previously written against overuse of Tamiflu, and especially against hording of it by patients, I was consciously reversing myself in a situation where I believed the drug to be useful. Andrew Pelletier, the head epidemiologist for the Maine division of the CDC, said that his caution was informed by federal directives. He was sympathetic to my view, while acknowledging that the Tamiflu protocol was based in part on fear of a shortage. Supplies in Maine were plentiful—the camp had been able to procure more than 400 courses of Tamiflu with ease. But the CDC was reluctant to dip too far into the supply, worried that not enough would be available if and when the new flu becomes more widespread (despite the fact that there were 50 million treatment courses of Tamiflu in the strategic national stockpile). As I had written, runs on Tamiflu and premature use of the drug, as people attempt to hoard it in case they or their families became sick, were another cause for concern.

With a vaccine not yet ready, using Tamiflu to control outbreaks at camps was exactly what I felt we should be doing. The chances of resistance developing from focused use of the drug to treat real outbreaks was quite small. The Maine CDC allowed Camp Modin to proceed, and the results were even more dramatic than I'd anticipated. Many studies examining control of the flu had used amantadine, an older antiviral drug, against the yearly flu. Camp Modin's experiment was perhaps the first in close quarters with Tamiflu against the new pandemic strain. When the camp started using it, the total number of cases was forty, and the daily incidence was fourteen. Two days later, the number of new cases was four. (See the Modin statistics) Though there were soon more than eighty campers and staff with the flu—all cases were mild, and the first three were confirmed as the H1N1 swine flu strain by the CDC—but no one on Tamiflu as a preventive measure became sick, not even the counselors and nurses who were caring for those in the quarantined area. While my son took his daily Tamiflu dose and enjoyed the wilds of Maine, the quarantined kids watched TV and played video games for a week before being allowed to return to their regular bunks. I couldn't tell whether Tamiflu prevented infection altogether or just kept kids from getting sick. But it didn't really matter. After a week, the camp collectively exhaled; the outbreak was over.

As cases of flu began to appear at other camps in Maine and around the United States (more than thirty summer camps in Maine and fifty in the United States were afflicted with H1N1 swine flu), word of Modin's successful containment spread, and pediatricians were again asked to fax prescriptions to Maine for Tamiflu. I published an account of the Modin outbreak in Slate, and Howard told me that camp directors throughout Maine were using the Modin Protocol to fuel and justify their own use of Tamiflu.

Camp Fernwood, with 330 campers and staff, quickly had twenty eight cases; a pregnant staff member isolated herself, while another, with a six month-old son, fled the camp. The camp director, Fritz Seving, adopted the Modin Protocol, and of 330 campers and staff, 297 took Tamiflu. (The suggested length of time for prophylaxis is seven days after being in contact with someone who has the flu.) Within a day of starting Tamiflu, Fernwood had no new cases, and the outbreak was quashed.

In establishing the Modin Protocol, I had spoken with Dr. Robert Press, our chief medical officer at NYU Langone Medical Center at the time and an infectious disease expert, and Dr. Michael Phillips, our main infectious disease epidemiologist at NYU Langone and Bellevue. Both agreed that Tamiflu could have a beneficial role in decreasing shedding time (being contagious) even in those with mild illness. Both also disagreed with the Maine CDC when it came to using Tamiflu prophylaxis on contacts during large outbreaks in camps. In fact, while I was advising Modin to give Tamiflu, Press was advising another camp in Maine to do the same.

But Dr. Martin Blaser, chairman of medicine at NYU Langone Medical Center at the timeand a world renowned infectious disease expert, didn't believe that quarantine and isolation were effective measures in the pandemic setting. "It is unrealistic," he said. "It is fine when there is an isolated outbreak. . . . Isn't it better to have the virus now, while it was still mild? What if it returned in a more severe form in the fall? Wouldn't I regret that my son and others at Modin hadn't had it?"

But thinking this point through, it was hard to justify deliberately exposing a child to infection in order to provoke immunization. That technique hadn't been used by public health officials since before the smallpox vaccine had been discovered. (Deliberate inoculation with smallpox, believed to have first been used in India in 1000 B.C. and famously employed by George Washington on troops during the Revolutionary War, has not been used since the late eighteenth century, when the smallpox vaccination was discovered.

Flash forward to 2020—I wonder what Dr. Blaser would say now about the COVID lockdowns—I hadn't had the opportunity to ask him yet.

The national CDC, had another concern that Dr. Blaser shared. They weren't in favor of the prophylactic use of Tamiflu. They agreed with Dr. Dora Anne Mills, Maine's public health director, who was concerned about resistance, and about it becoming a trend. And at a press conference on July 23, Dr. Anne Schuchat, director of the National Center on Immunization and Respiratory Diseases at the CDC, said she "strongly recommended" giving Tamiflu only to those who were seriously ill or their contacts who had chronic illnesses.

Camp Modin's director, Howard Salzberg, continued to believe he had done the right thing, following my reasoning that the camp environment was similar to health care centers and nursing homes, and that this time it was the kids rather than the elderly who were most at risk. I agreed with Dr. Blaser that isolation was almost impossible, but I ultimately disagreed with him about Tamiflu. It was a difficult decision, but on balance, the best argument was that judicious use for large outbreaks could help to decrease circulating virus while we waited for the vaccine. If Modin had closed, which was likely without Tamiflu, H1N1 would have been spread to many zip codes as well as to Europe, where several of the counselors and campers originated.

It also wasn't clear that a shortage was a realistic concern. The CDC had already stockpiled 50 million courses of Tamiflu, with more to follow. Tamiflu might be less necessary as a preventive once a vaccine was being commonly used. But in advance of a vaccine, Tamiflu was an effective way to quash H1N1 outbreaks and protect the most vulnerable. If we used it properly now, we might not need it as much in the future. I still believed it was time for the CDC to change its protocol, though I knew they wouldn't.

MODIN STATISTICS

- 16 new cases of the influenza H1N1 swine flu strain, June 24–29
- 24 new cases on June 30
- Tamiflu treatment and prophylaxis started on July 1 and 2
- 14 new cases on July 1
- 15 new cases on July 2
- 4 new cases on July 3
- 3 new cases on July 4
- 1 new case on July 5
- 1 new case on July 6
- 0 new cases on July 7
- 6,000 screening temperatures taken
- 5 children stopped Tamiflu due to nausea.
- Children were screened by the camp doctor, Dr. Marvin Lee, for ear, sinus, and throat infections that often accompany the flu, and antibiotics were prescribed for four children.

AUGUST 2009

As the new H1N1 swine flu strain continued to spread through July in the Southern Hemisphere (in Chile, 99 percent of the circulating flu was the new H1N1 strain, whereas in Australia it was mixed with a seasonal H3N2 strain), preparations continued for a massive vaccination program to commence sometime in October. In the meantime, there were close to 500 more deaths, mostly in Argentina, Chile, and Brazil. Symptoms remained similar to the seasonal flu, with fever, fatigue, cough, headache, muscle aches, sore throat, and runny nose. Diarrhea and vomiting were sometimes seen. Most cases remained mild. In the United States by the end of July, 5,414 people had required hospitalization, with 353 deaths, but there were believed to be well over 1 million cases by this point. By August 1 there were 186,720 confirmed cases in the world (there were several million unconfirmed cases), with 1,404 deaths.

On July 30, a British study was released that threw a slight wrench into my thinking about Tamiflu. Published in Eurosurveillance, the study looked at 103 students at a London school who received Tamiflu as a precaution after a classmate received a diagnosis of swine flu. Of those taking Tamiflu, 45 experienced one or more side effects most completely GI symptoms, followed by thinking problems. Though previous studies (mainly in adults) had shown nausea as a fairly common side effect, the neuropsychiatric disturbance was believed to be very rare. At Camp Modin, where more than 300 campers and 130 staff had taken the drug, there were only five cases of nausea. At Camp Fernwood, the drug was equally well tolerated.

In early August, an Oxford University study published in the British Medical Journal reviewed the data from four other randomized studies involving 1,766 children and found little effect in preventing secondary complications such as asthma or ear infections, with twice as much risk of developing nausea (up to 20 percent of patients).

These studies were at odds with previous studies as well as our effective results at Modin. By contrast, the Modin and Fernwood data were based on twenty-four hour surveillance of patients and contacts and were only H1N1 swine flu. It was clear speaking to Howard Salzberg that the Modin results were dramatically different from the British data. "We saw very little nausea or intolerance," he said. "I estimate that no more than five people stopped taking the Tamiflu out of four hundred."

THE VACCINE

In late July, as America woke up to the possibility of a strong return and expansion of the H1N1 swine flu in the fall and winter, stories and questions about the new vaccine emerged in the news media. Why is it taking so long? Will I have to take one shot or two? Will it contain mercury (thimerosal)? Who should take it?

The answers to these questions also emerged. The vaccine was taking so long because most of the manufacturers (including Sanofi Pasteur, Baxter, and GSK) were using the old 1950s-style hen egg medium to culture the virus. Harvesting billions of hen eggs took months. Only one manufacturer, Novartis, was using the newer mammalian egg technology, where the virus is grown in cell culture, similar to the way that the hepatitis and other new vaccines are grown. Novartis had started their clinical trials in July. Overall there were twenty four clinical trials ongoing throughout July, all involving dead virus, with the exception of Medimmune's weakened live virus vaccine (it is squirted into the nose and cannot be used in patients with lung disease or those who are immuno compromised).

A small company named Protein Sciences Corp., based in Connecticut, had received a $35 million grant from the Department of Health and Human Services to pursue new technology for a novel H1N1 swine flu vaccine. The company was producing a hundred thousand doses of vaccine per week using caterpillar ovary cells and an insect virus (baculovirus) that doesn't harm humans.

With nine of the twenty four clinical trials involving more traditional methods completed by the end of July, discussion began in earnest about who should be vaccinated and when. A fifteen member CDC panel identified those at highest risk who needed the vaccine the most. Pregnant women were at the top of the list, because a recent survey showed that 6 percent of the people who died with the new strain were pregnant. This made sense, since pregnancy is a period of compromised immunity. The CDC panel also recommended that health care workers be vaccinated, which also made sense, since we would be at the front lines treating those with flu. Of course, older people with chronic illnesses were included. But what was dramatically different from the yearly flu recommendations was the targeting of children for vaccination.

This was appropriate. First, children had the worst cases. Second, flu spreads easily at schools. In Japan, flu vaccination for schoolchildren was mandatory for most of twenty five years beginning in the 1960s, and a study in the New England Journal of Medicine in 2001 confirmed that Japan had experienced more than a million less deaths from all causes during this time.

Kids are superspreaders of flu, and if an effective children's vaccination program for the new strain could be successfully completed, a herd immunity could be established, and the new flu would be dealt a serious blow. The CDC's new director, Dr. Tom Frieden, announced in early August that the CDC would urge schools to stay open in the fall unless so many kids were sick that the school could no longer function, or if parents persisted in sending sick kids knowingly to school (as had happened at Camp Modin).

In the meantime, the vaccine was coming along more slowly than many experts hoped. It definitely wouldn't be ready for the start of school. Using the old technology for most of the batch would certainly be useful to reassure people that the vaccine was safe, but it meant that we wouldn't be seeing it until late October, when 40 million doses were expected to be ready, and mid November, when an additional 120 million doses would follow. A total of 160 million doses would be just enough to cover the risk groups listed above, with healthy adults to follow as more vaccine became available in November.

To make matters worse, the WHO announced in early August that the swine flu strain wasn't growing well in chicken eggs, which could delay production further. It also wasn't clear yet how effective the vaccine was going to be. For years I and others had been publicly urging the transition from the old egg vaccine to a more modern vaccine to try out with the yearly flu so it would be ready for use in a pandemic. Now it was too late. It was likely that a more modern vaccine would be more effective, but we would never know. Patients could receive the swine flu vaccine at the same time as they had their yearly flu vaccine, but children and those in high-risk groups might need a booster shot to the swine flu inoculation three weeks later. The results of clinical trials would determine if this was necessary. If we could only manage to vaccinate most of the world's population (a herculean task), we could see the new pandemic slow. Since pandemics don't follow strict seasons and tend to stretch on for years, vaccination could play a crucial role in slowing spread. There was bound to be a great deal of fear and non-compliance to deal with when the vaccine came out.

PANDEMIC PRECAUTIONS

I had been treating dozens of patients for this flu in my office all spring, and as time went on, my own fears lessened. At first, back in April and May, I was literally afraid to examine a patient with flu, afraid that I would bring it home to my children. But as I saw case after case without getting sick, I began to relax. Perhaps I was immune.

The symptoms varied from one patient to the next but generally included fatigue, fever, muscle aches, sore throat, headache, and sometimes nausea—very similar to the yearly flu only milder, and not lasting as long.

A study from Hong Kong, published in the Annals of Internal Medicine in early August, appeared to show that early use of masks and careful hand-washing could significantly decrease the spread of influenza within a household. This was still a controversial area; it clearly applied only to people who had the flu, not to the general public walking down the street. There was no value to wearing a mask in public if you weren't sick; of course this recommendation would change dramatically ten years later for a different respiratory virus which launched the kind of pandemic that was as comparable to the 2009 pandemic as a shark was to a goldfish.

Another public health concern come fall would be the hospitals. If fear made a comeback, and sniffling worriers once again began to clog the emergency rooms, these places would soon become incapable of taking care of those who were really sick, from flu as well as other ailments. We didn't have the surge capacity in our hospitals in the United States to handle a real pandemic; we didn't have the emergency room space to handle either excess illness or fear of illness. This too was to become extremely problematic in the Spring and Summer of 2020.

Back in 2009, we had the Tamiflu but we lacked the vaccines. We also lacked the antibiotics to treat all the pneumonias that could result. We didn't have the respirators we needed for the very ill. Most of all, we lacked the ability to deal with our own fear of the unknown.

Businesses and schools began to put together pandemic protocols, contingency plans that would attempt to account for absences and no shows, both from the flu as well as the need to be a caretaker if your children got the flu. Fear of the flu also would keep many home unnecessarily if media hype and fear mongering spiraled out of control, as I expected it would. Public health announcements and press conferences stressing the worst case scenario would likely resurface as soon as the fall arrived and there were a new handful of swine flu deaths.

In the meantime, there was a lingering public complacency even while some businesses and schools got ready. Hand wipes were purchased, hand-washing was stressed, common surfaces were disinfected. Plans were made to use skeleton crews and to work in shifts to minimize contact. Working from home via computer was considered as a viable option.

It was important to stay home with the flu, I counseled many businesses; otherwise it would spread until the school or business would have to close. Luckily, the pandemic looked like it would still be quite mild, as pandemics went. Perhaps this was the reason for complacency alternating with fear —the terms "mild" and "pandemic" didn't combine in a way people could easily understand.

But this complacency could quickly fade; as fall approached and we anticipated the early flu season that was characteristic of pandemics, I was most concerned that if our public health authorities began to have press conferences and if the news media once again attached their giant megaphone, the risks of the flu would be surpassed by the fear that accompanied it. People who were very afraid not only clogged emergency rooms, they also took fewer precautions and tended not to listen to advice.

In August, 2009, the CDC reported that the rapid test for flu (nasal swab) was only 40 to 69 percent sensitive to the new strain, based on a test of 65 people. The test was only positive when there was a lot of virus in the sample, which means the best time to test people was in the first days after they became symptomatic and were shedding the most virus.

For practicing doctors like me, this meant that I wouldn't rely completely on a test result, and for a patient with flu symptoms at this odd time of the year for flu, I would assume they had swine flu and start them on Tamiflu right away, especially if they were pregnant, had another illness, or had a bad case of the flu.

THE FLU PROPHET

Lone Simonsen is one of the world's top experts in infectious disease epidemiology and pandemics. She has been a senior adviser to the NIH, the CDC, and the WHO for many years. Simonsen has written extensively about prior flu pandemics, describing them as characterized by a shift in virus subtypes, shifts of higher death rates to younger populations, successive waves, higher transmissibility than the yearly flu, and different impacts depending on geographic region (the new swine flu virus had appeared more severe in Mexico in the spring, and in certain parts of South America in July and August).

In any pandemic, Simonsen emphasized when we spoke, even a mild one, the death toll depended on the rapidity of preventive and therapeutic measures, including social distancing and the treatment of secondary infections, especially pneumonia.

She said she believed in the use of the rapid influenza test to help public health officials to separate flu from other respiratory illnesses. She also believed in using blood tests (serology) to see who was immune among those who were exposed. "I would be very pleased to find out I already had it myself," she said, though she acknowledged that this new flu lacked the virulence markers of previous pandemics and could well remain quite mild.

Simonsen agreed with me that we needed to rethink how we used Tamiflu prophylaxis, in terms of having "more respect for resistant strains" as well as for "prudent blocking" of transmission and to snuff out outbreaks, as I had suggested at Camp Modin. "But there is no need to go all out with Tamiflu right now," she said.

Simonsen also believed that the number of H1N1 swine flu cases was being drastically underestimated by the CDC and the WHO, and that most influenza like illness in the late spring and summer had in fact been from the new swine flu. She agreed with me that the WHO lacked a coordinated response or an effective definition of pandemic that encompassed both the extent and the severity of the virus.

The WHO would show the same type of fumbling ten years later, though for political reasons that went beyond simple ineptitude.

As we looked toward the fall, Simonsen predicted a resurgence. She was cautious about the upcoming vaccine and reflected on the 1976 swine flu vaccine, which had been hastily given and had seemingly led to the side effect of Guillain Barré syndrome. She felt it could have been due to the impurity of the vaccine or giving it in conjunction with the seasonal flu vaccine. She was concerned again now about the rare possibility of antibodies developing against peripheral nerves but waved that off because there was a real pandemic to fight, albeit a mild one.

Simonsen felt that the more modern cell culture vaccine that Novartis was making should be "rushed through" and be considered for the "prevailing vaccine."

In fact their vaccine would receive extensive use, along with vaccines made by CSL Limited, Sanofi Pasteur, and a nasal-spray vaccine produced by MedImmune.

Simonsen predicted that this pandemic would extend over a few years and be mild to moderate, just as the previous two had in the 1950s and 1960s. But vaccines could make a real difference this time, whereas they had played a lesser role during the prior two pandemics. She ended up being 100 percent correct, as usual. Like me, Simonsen was a big proponent of vaccinating everyone to "decrease the amount of circulating virus." Healthy people, she said, could receive the live virus mist, and the elderly should all be vaccinated as part of any effective immunization strategy. This also ended up being the direction we would take.

Lone Simonsen, flu strategist, expert, and prophet all rolled into one, said with a sigh into the phone from Washington, D.C., "We must take it seriously. It is a pandemic, but it is much less of a risk than 1918, at least so far. We have to stay ahead of it as best we can, and to use vaccines more effectively than we have before."

A pandemic, but much less of a risk than 1918, and also the one to come next.

LATE AUGUST 2009: THE PRESIDENT'S COUNCIL OF ADVISORS

As the flu season ended in the Southern Hemisphere, it had clearly been a heavy season but not an overwhelming one. Most patients recovered without treatment and were only mildly ill. The WHO raised some eyebrows with the statement that in some areas there appeared to be a more severe form that caused more respiratory complications, but careful genetic tracking continued to show no sign that the virus was mutating into a more severe strain. As with previous pandemics, swine flu was twenty times more common in the five to-twenty-four year old age group and was initially killing mostly people in their twenties, thirties, and forties. But the overall death toll remained very very low—still less than 2,500 cases worldwide as we reached the end of August.

Nevertheless, a draconian planning scenario issued by the president's Council of Advisors on Science and Technology in late August suddenly predicted that we could see half the U.S. population become infected with the H1N1 swine flu virus, leading to 1.8 million hospitalizations with 30,000 to 90,000 deaths. This report immediately elicited a worried response. For one thing, American hospitals, which were more than 80 percent filled on average, and overflowing in many cases, were hardly ready for the kind of surge in need that these numbers predicted. There was a shortage of respirators, emergency rooms, and even intravenous antibiotics to treat secondary pneumonias.

Panic could easily become the greatest public health concern. If these numbers took hold, worried snifflers would once again be clogging the emergency rooms, interfering with the need to take care of our sickest patients who didn't have the flu.

Fear was also a concern in our businesses and schools. In late August, the flu continued to spread predominantly among colleges that began to return to session. Fear soon replaced complacency on campuses. It was clear that the new strain of flu was still spreading mostly among children and young adults, who lacked immunity to it. The University of Alabama reported fifty four cases on its first day of classes. Close to sixty cases were reported by Louisiana State University sororities. Duke University had an outbreak among its football team during the preseason. The outbreaks were small and mild, but fear was building as the outbreaks were timed to the council's report.

The threat of economic ruin if businesses and schools were disrupted by absences and panic (the CDC was suggesting not closing schools this time) was reminiscent of SARS. Back in 2003, SARS had infected 8,400 people, killing 774 worldwide, with 33 probable U.S. cases but no deaths. After analyzing all the data from this outbreak (initially projected as far worse), the WHO finally concluded that SARS is not spread easily through the air.

Yet while the science was still in question, fear driven responses had led to travel advisories in Asia and at least $30 billion in lost revenues to local economies. Toronto also was isolated by virtue of public health travel restrictions, and billions of Canadian dollars were lost there as well.

The new planning scenario for H1N1 swine flu, based as it was on past pandemics, was likely to provoke fear and overreaction, suggesting that these lessons had not been properly learned with SARS. The last flu pandemic, in 1968, did kill 33,000 in the United States, but that was around the same amount as for the yearly flu, and the current H1N1 virus seemed much milder. For the millions around the world who had already been infected, there had only been just over two thousand deaths by the end of

August. Granted, pandemics tend to worsen over time, and granted, they tend to be extended over more than one flu season, but even taking this into account, the council's projections of infections, hospitalizations, and deaths still appeared way overblown.

There was some concern that the president's Council of Advisors on Science and Technology might have been motivated by the need to justify funding for the swine flu response. Though co chairs Dr. James Holdren (environmentalist and policy expert at the Kennedy School of Government) and Dr. Eric Lander (director of the Broad Institute at MIT and a leader in the human genome project), and Dr. Harold Varmus, CEO of Memorial Sloan Kettering Cancer Center and former head of the NIH, were all notable scientists, none of them had expertise in flu. The fact that they were leading the way with their projected numbers was even more problematic given their lack of expertise. Many critics even wondered if the Obama administration would use the scary projection as a justification for the health reform bill.

Whereas I was mostly concerned that the fear generated could cripple our emergency response system for a novel virus that was spreading extensively but that was likely to remain mild and lead to far fewer hospitalizations (except from fear) and deaths than the president's advisors anticipated.

My view ended up being prescient, when you consider how wholly unprepared we were for COVID-19

SEPTEMBER 2009

As school began, there were several outbreaks of H1N1 swine flu around the country, especially in the Southeast. The WHO suggested that if schools decided to close, they should do so early in an outbreak for the best result at controlling spread.

With the H1N1 swine flu vaccine not expected to be widely available for at least two more months, clinical trials continued to show that it was well tolerated, and a new study published in the New England Journal of Medicine revealed that only one shot was needed to provide immunity in adults. The dose necessary was 15 mcg (same as for the yearly flu vaccine), and immunity was achieved in eight to ten days. This was a very exciting and effective result.

EBOLA: OUTBREAKS IN AFRICA CAUSE PANIC HERE

In the summer of 2020 a new outbreak of 100 plus cases of Ebola in a western province the Democratic Republic of Congo (43 patients died) had doubled in just five weeks and public health officials were concerned. The World Health Organization pledged $2.5 million to help control the outbreak, but the Congo Health Ministry said that $40 million was needed and the rest of the world was focused on the coronavirus pandemic. Congo just completed fighting an Ebola outbreak in its eastern provinces that killed 2,200 people.

Merck's new Ebola vaccine has been effective in helping to overcome the outbreak, with more than 250,000 people receiving it. A stockpile of 500,000 doses of Ebola vaccines (beginning with this one) is now being established by GAVI, the global vaccine and immunization alliance, with plans for poorer countries to be able to have it without charge.

2014

The 2019–20 Ebola outbreaks still weren't of the order of the 2014-15 West Africa urban outbreak that killed more than 11,300 people and spread to other countries in the world including the U.S.

But as deadly as Ebola is, it is not very contagious, so it is much more easily contained than a virus like SARS COV2. Because of how deadly it is (more than 50 percent mortality in many regions), the fear quotient is very high, and in 2014 it was a "bug du jour" here in the U.S. despite very few cases.

The Ebola virus had been infecting and killing people in Central Africa since at least 1976, and the 2014 "worst Ebola epidemic in history" had been going on for several months. But then another virus emerged, the virus of fear.

Don't get me wrong, Ebola was a bad bug, and well worth being concerned about. But it was not very contagious. It often fooled the immune system of a host into not recognizing it, and many victims ended up in kidney and liver failure without even a fight. On top of this, Ebola was difficult to recognize, appearing first like any other flu with fatigue, fever, headache, muscle aches. Then you could start to have vomiting and diarrhea, and caretakers and close contacts of afflicted patients could catch Ebola even as they tried to help contain it.

But fear and ignorance was spreading in West Africa along with Ebola in 2014, as natives mistrusted the very humanitarian aid that was being brought in to help them. Physicians in the Ebola trenches were heroes, not sources of contagion, but not everyone saw them that way. Dr. Sheik Humarr Khan, whose work in Sierra Leone against several viruses -- including Ebola -- was legendary, died in 2014 while battling Ebola.

Isolating sick patients and their contacts worked in stopping Ebola outbreaks. The same kind of infection-control precautions were used that had also worked successfully with HIV/AIDS (gloves, gowns, masks).

Unfortunately, when people were afraid, they took fewer infectious precautions, and spread more virus.

The challenge to provide supportive care while properly isolating patients was much greater in Liberia, Sierra Leone, or Guinea than it would be here.

Living close together, being unaware of how viruses spread, and even burial rituals helped to spread Ebola in West Africa. Fear was the operative term as villagers feared the Red Cross and Doctors Without Borders and associated them with the virus. Natives trusted their local medicine men.

But the virus remained difficult to contract. Thomas Duncan the Liberian patient who died in Dallas, was in touch with 100 people after his arrival in the U.S. and none of them got sick.

Doctors on the front lines in Africa showed courage in the face of the disease and were inspiring role models.

By late December 2014, Dr. Kombu Songu-M'briwa had recovered enough from his personal battle with Ebola to participate in a transatlantic radio interview with me, though I could barely hear him because of the profound fatigue reflected in his voice.

M'briwa, one of just three doctors working at the 120-bed Hastings Ebola treatment center in Freetown, Sierra Leone, told me that early identification of his infection in late November, replacing fluids and treating accompanying infections with antibiotics had been the key to his recovery. This was in keeping with the latest statistics from the region, where survival rates had finally now reached 70 percent.

Shielded by his new immunity and returning courage, M'briwa said he would go back into the community to help educate the people there, as well as to identify and isolate new cases. He was one of the great heroes in the fight against Ebola.

The population's response in Sierra Leone was not yet at the level of Liberia, where infection rates had dropped by 80 percent.

"Community mobilization occurred in Liberia due to local volunteers, women's groups, youth groups and the participation of faith communities, [and] has been highly effective," explained Dr. Timothy Flanigan, professor of infectious diseases at the Warren Alpert Medical School of Brown University as well as a permanent deacon and volunteer with the Catholic Church's Ebola Response Team.

Flanigan provided guidance and safety at Liberian health facilities. "Ebola causes such intense fear because it is such a dreadful virus," he said. "I developed great admiration for the nurses and staff in the clinics that stayed open despite the fear."

The chain of transmission was broken in Liberia by basic public health measures: isolating the sick, burying the dead safely and quarantining those who were exposed. The presence of the U.S. military brought needed resources: more treatment centers and helicopters to transport patients and supplies.

Ebola had a major impact on the health care infrastructure in the affected countries of West Africa. Dr. Estrella Lasry, who had been in the field for months as the tropical medicine adviser for Doctors Without Borders, told me she was concerned about the disease's burgeoning impact on malaria and other tropical illnesses. At the same time, care for non-communicable diseases like heart disease and cancer had been drastically diminished, and essentials such as prenatal care and childhood vaccinations were difficult to come by, much as has happened now worldwide during the coronavirus pandemic.

By some estimates, over 10,000 children have been orphaned by Ebola. At the same time, care for children with Ebola was especially difficult.

"You see kids suffering Ebola, they just don't feel well, they want to be touched, they want to be hugged," said Marina Novack, a nurse with Doctors Without Borders who recently returned from Sierra Leone said to me in an interview.

"When you're wearing a PPE (Personal Protective Equipment), you are scary-looking to them, they still want you to hold them and they reach for you. But because there is the risk that one of them may knock off your goggles or rip your gloves, you're unable to carry them."

Since the outbreak began in March, 2014, Doctors Without Borders played a prominent role, admitting more than 7,000 patients to its facilities, with more than 4,000 confirmed as having Ebola. More than 1,300 tons of supplies had been shipped to the affected countries, but Director Sophie Delaunay told me the needs were constantly changing, because Ebola was a moving target.

Unfortunately, there were too many instances of helicopters dedicated to transporting single vials of blood or ferrying specimens instead of infected patients.

Delaunay echoed Flanigan's sentiment that coordination of services remained crucial to controlling the outbreak. Furthermore, she said, "It's essential, in addition to the isolation units, to be able to provide the full package of education, awareness raising, safe burial, contact training and surveillance"—actions that allowed relative success to be achieved in Liberia. Virus hunter Joseph Fair, special adviser to Sierra Leone's health ministry, had been on the front lines for months, and he correctly predicted many more months would pass before they could turn the corner on the epidemic.

Still, he said, there had been significant improvements in awareness in Sierra Leone. "We went from half the population believing that this wasn't a real disease and was a possible hoax to everyone more or less believing that this is a real disease and learning how it is transmitted," he told me. "It's really helping stabilize the spread, along with open beds."

Fair added that the unprecedented number of cases had allowed for a more detailed study of the disease and treatments. It was no more transmissible than originally thought but was more of a gastrointestinal virus, he said.

Here in the U.S., where hysteria had been the operative term and only four cases had been diagnosed and 10 cases treated, Dr. Michael Phillips, infectious disease specialist and director of the infection prevention and control unit at NYU Langone Medical Center, told me that the keys to restoring public confidence were protocol and preparation.

This was evidenced in October by his expert management of the treatment given Dr. Craig Spencer at Bellevue Hospital Center, where a highly coordinated team approach led to a positive outcome without spread. The Spencer case ultimately helped to calm public fears, though the CDC bungling of an Ebola specimen, putting a lab worker at risk, again threatened to weaken public confidence.

I was outside Bellevue Hospital with a camera crew, reporting for Megyn Kelly and *The Kelly File* on the admission of Craig Spencer to Bellevue. I reassured the viewers that Bellevue had a long history as a quarantine center and was well equipped to handle this without it spreading. I turned out to be right.

A few days later I boarded a Frontier Airlines plane with the CEO and sat in the same seat that Amber Vinson, a nurse from Dallas who had contracted Ebola, had sat. Once again I was able to reassure viewers that I was completely unconcerned about the casual spread of Ebola. My goal was to calm public fears.

Phillips said he believed it was "normal for emerging diseases to scare us because they are unknown," but at the same time we had to learn to overcome these fears and focus our attention on the real problem in West Africa.

His wise observation remained as true in 2020 as it was back in 2014, when Ebola fighters were designated Time Magazine's Person of the Year for 2014, an honor they richly deserved.

Dr. M'Briwa was simultaneously one of the fighters and one of the victims. Once recovered, as fighter once again, he continued to push forward to bring an end to this crisis in his native Sierra Leone.

Might his courage back then serve as an inspiration to all of us now, in the fight against COVID-19.

ZIKA:
FACTS AND FEARS

FEBRUARY 2016

Back in February, 2016, I spoke this week with a pregnant woman who had just returned from Mexico. She wasn't feeling ill; she was visiting the obstetrics facility at New York University for a screening ultrasound of her fetus. There is no instinct stronger than that of a woman protecting her unborn child, and this woman was nervous because she was unable to obtain a rapid Zika test (only an ultrasound at the time) to relieve her fears. She said the Zika virus was now just one more danger she had to worry about.

At the time, the Zika virus (carried by the Aedes mosquito), and Zika fears were just beginning to spread in the U.S. Governor Rick Scott of Florida declared a state of emergency in four counties over nine cases ,fanning the fear flames

On the same day, a case surfaced of a patient in Texas who reportedly became infected with Zika through sexual contact, and suddenly there were medical warnings to use condoms or abstain from sex with travelers from the region. Dr. Tom Frieden, then director of the Centers for Disease Control, reassured me in an interview that the risk of sexual transmission was extremely low, and Dr. Anthony Fauci, director of the National Institute for Allergy and Infectious Diseases, told me he didn't expect Zika to become widespread in the U.S.

So why were we so afraid of Zika?

For one thing, the name sounded exotic and mysterious, like a killer from a faraway place. For another, we had never heard of it until January, 2016, and we were naturally afraid of something unknown or new—especially when it was something we couldn't control.

Zika was soon put under the microscope of the news media and the World Health Organization, which conducted meetings and issued ominous warnings, and this sudden public health focus alarmed us. A survey conducted by travel risk manager On Call International found that 64 percent of Americans who responded, whether they were pregnant or not, said they would cancel their trips to affected areas.

We saw images of infants with tiny heads and undersized brains, and they understandably petrified us. Of the 3 million live births in 2015 in Brazil, more than 4,000 were reported—and 270 were confirmed—to have the terrible birth defect microcephaly, or small head. In a typical year, there are just over 100 cases. Frieden said at the time Zika's exact role in these cases had yet to be determined (it was later proven to be the cause), and the CDC was working closely with Brazilian health authorities.

We heard about rare cases of Guilliain-Barre Syndrome (ascending paralysis) being associated with Zika, and we worried about that too.

We learned that Zika had no symptoms 80 percent of the time, which should have reassured us, but it actually made things worse. Nothing scares people more than an invisible danger.

Travel advisories made sense, but the need for them inflated the perception that simply traveling south puts you at risk. No public health official wanted to be responsible for even one horrible birth defect, but the perception of risk was far greater than the reality for Zika in 2016.

As with all health scares, we had to do our best to counter worry with information and perspective. Fauci was reassuring when he told me that we could win the worldwide battle with the mosquito, that Brazil had effectively curtailed the problem before, only to see the Aedes Aegypti mosquito (which carries Dengue as well as Zika) swarm back when public health measures—including using larvicides and insecticides and ridding public places of still water—went lax.

A more rational focus on the Zika virus alerted us to the need for greater focus on global health concerns that involved mosquito vectors. The Aedes Aegypti mosquito carried Dengue, Yellow Fever, Chikungunya and Zika. It was a massive killer of humans worldwide, and we needed a coordinated campaign to wipe it out. Public health also needed far more financial support for vaccine research. Fauci told me that the NIH was accelerating work on a Zika vaccine (it was still in development in 2020), and he expected one to be commercially available in two to three years.

The sudden spread of Zika was concerning, but the fear of it was worse. To provide perspective to fight the fear we needed to know more than just the numerator, the number of cases of microcephaly that could result. We needed to know the denominator, the number of total cases, because the vast majority had no problem at all.

APRIL 2016

When it comes to an emerging contagion, it's often difficult for the news media to deliver a balanced message. Inflammatory health scares are partly the fault of a public health official presenting a skewed version of the facts but on top of this the media megaphones said "facts" and uses the official for hyped soundbites.

Never was that truer than with the rise of the Zika virus in the Americas. With Zika, it was hard to comprehend the extent of the threat because it is a virus that causes little or no symptoms in the vast majority of people who acquire it from a mosquito bite, and yet at the same time it carries the rare risk of birth defects, especially those involving the brain. Pictures of afflicted babies were what garnered attention, not the multitude of Zika sufferers who got better without complications.

Dr. Fauci repeatedly attempted to deliver nuanced messages about Zika—and for the most part, he did so effectively. Unfortunately, in April, 2016, when he said he expected limited outbreaks in the U.S. this summer, all anyone heard was the wordoutbreak. But Fauci told me in an interview that the problem and solution both lay in mosquito control: There could not be a widespread outbreak unless the virus took hold in the local Aedes aegypti mosquito population, and he did not expect that to happen. He pointed to evidence that a related virus, dengue—carried by the same mosquito—had become widespread in other parts of the world but never here in the U.S.

Fauci supported President Obama's $1.9 billion proposal to Congress to fight Zika. He said that without this allocation, money would have to be taken from other budgets to cover costs for the fight against Zika, which could lead to underfunding. There was also the need for funding for the ongoing promising vaccine research. (In late September $1.1 billion was finally approved by Congress)

Zika was first discovered in Uganda in the 1940s but it was only in 2016 that it was considered by international public health officials to be more than a nuisance virus. This was prompted by the epidemic in Brazil, and throughout Central America and the Caribbean, where the culprit mosquito was plentiful. But of course the obsessive focus was fueled because the risk to unborn children has yet to be quantified, both in terms of time of greatest susceptibility, and extent and frequency of brain injury. Not knowing the extent of a risk spreads uncertainty—which spreads fear. People who are afraid personalize the risk and believe they are bound to be the virus's next victim, whether they are pregnant or not. It is too easy to forget that 80 percent of the time Zika causes no symptoms, and that no one dies from it. Dr. Fauci became our main fear guide with Zika, understanding that worry over the virus was contagious even though the virus almost never was. Fauci did his best to adjust his public health messaging to adequately address both problems. Unfortunately, it was much more difficult for him to communicate anti-fear sound-bite messages with COVID, in 2020, a far more dangerous and highly contagious virus.

MAY 2016

Eighty years prior to the summer of 2016, courageous people from all over the world travelled to Berlin for the Nazi-hosted Olympics, none more famously than Jesse Owens. It was ironic that as this event was being commemorated, the upcoming Olympics in Brazil were in danger of being cancelled due to fear.

It was the fear of Zika, not the threat of the virus itself, that was causing some people to call for delaying, moving, or cancelling the Rio games. One proponent of postponement, relocation, or both was University of Ottawa professor Amir Attaran, who suggested proceeding as planned could create "a full-blown global health disaster."

At the same time, Major League Baseball relocated a series between the Pirates and the Marlins originally scheduled to be held in Puerto Rico, which seems an overreaction now, looking back at it from the vantage point of a true pandemic.

Fear kept people from remembering that almost all Zika transmission required a mosquito—particularly an infected female of an Aedes species. (While sexual transmission of Zika is possible, wearing condoms was an effective way to stop the spread of the disease – and even the Pope agreed it was the right move.)

And though the U.S. has the right mosquitoes (Aedes aegypti), it is extremely unlikely that we will ever have a Zika epidemic. Dengue fever, which is transmitted by the same mosquito, has never taken root here, despite more than 200,000 cases a year in neighboring Mexico, for example.

LESS RISK

The U.S. didn't have the same kind of mosquito-control problem that Brazil had, even in poorer areas where there was a lot of still water. *Aedes* mosquitoes typically lay eggs in and near standing water in things like buckets, bowls, animal dishes, flower pots and vases. They are aggressive daytime biters, prefer to bite people, and live indoors and outdoors near people.

The number of Zika cases reported in Brazil increased dramatically in 2016, with more than 90,000 likely cases registered by the Brazilian health ministry from February to the beginning of April.

And yes, 35,505 of these cases were in the Olympic city of Rio de Janeiro, while there had also been 4,908 cases of confirmed or suspected associated microcephaly. But for most people, Zika remained very mild or asymptomatic.

FLAMES OF FEAR

On the other hand, scientists continued fanning the fear flames with grandiose statements. Attaran wrote of a scenario in which "an estimated 500,000 foreign tourists flock into Rio for the Games, potentially becoming infected, and returning to their homes where both local *Aedes* mosquitoes and sexual transmission can establish new outbreaks".

In the light of such proclamations, the WHO's response (a joint statement with the Pan American Health Organization) that "the Games will take place during Brazil's wintertime, when the risk of being bitten is lower" did not reassure panicked travellers. On the other hand, it ended up being correct, as the case numbers fell before the Olympics took place.

And a study from the University of California at Berkeley a year later revealed that not a single case of Zika could be linked to the Olympics themselves. The cases were urban and local and the truly vulnerable were the city's lower socioeconomic groups as was so often the case.

AUGUST 18TH, 2016

Over the summer, the news about Zika continued to inflame and fright people. An infant born in Texas died due to complications from microcephaly, the first death in Texas to have resulted from Zika. Local transmission continued in Florida: The state began to offer free testing to pregnant women, a critically important step, but federal funding was still missing. Fear mongering continued. A Guardian piece speculated that an outbreak could be "bigger than we know," because we weren't doing extensive testing in other places where the disease may occur.

Puerto Rico was a different story and had over 5,000 cases. Zika was new to the U.S., but we knew how to contain it. This was because we'd fought the battle against its host, the Aedes aegypti mosquito, many times before and won.

The fight was waged in the past not because of Zika, but because of two far more severe viruses this mosquito could also transmit: Dengue fever and yellow fever.

In 1793, several thousand people died of yellow fever in Philadelphia, famously forcing George Washington to move the U.S. capital. In 1828, the disease moved south to New Orleans and settled in along the Mississippi River. Memphis, Tennessee, alone had six major yellow fever outbreaks in the 19th century, the last causing 2,000 cases and 600 deaths in 1879. But in 1901, mosquito control efforts began, and the last U.S. outbreak occurred in 1905 in New Orleans. Furthermore, a very effective vaccine became available in 1930.

The other Aedes aegypti–carried disease is Dengue fever (also known as "breakbone fever" because it may include severe joint and muscle aches), which had been infecting humans since 1789. According to the World Health Organization, as of 2016 the disease still caused 400 million cases globally each year. There was a new Dengue vaccine, Dengvaxia, becoming readily available which was also controversial because it could increase the risk of severe infection in some people.

Here in the U.S., outbreaks of Dengue were sporadic (and smaller—the largest since World War II occurred in Hawaii in 2015 and infected just 150 people, while most outbreaks infected less than 50).

It was because of Dengue that this country's public health officials figured out how to control Aedes aegypti, the disease-carrying mosquito that lives in coastal areas during the summer months. We did that with Naled, an insecticide that is almost 100 percent fatal for the Aedes aegypti mosquito.

The chemical was already sprayed on about 16 million acres a year in the continental U.S., according to the Centers for Disease Control and Prevention and the Environmental Protection Agency. The other measure that helped reduce these populations was the removal of standing water, since that's where mosquitos breed

Zika was expected to follow the same course of isolated sporadic outbreaks as Dengue because it was transmitted by the same mosquito. By August 2020 Florida had 33 cases of locally acquired Zika, most of them in a 1-square-mile area in Miami's Wynwood neighborhood. This looked very similar to what a small Dengue outbreak would look like, with comparable numbers. Wynwood might have been the epicenter because there was a lot of standing water in the area, and mosquitoes could easily breed there. That's why the CDC was targeting that neighborhood with Naled, to kill adult mosquitos, and a larvicide—which had been effective at reducing mosquito populations. Of course, these small outbreaks would continue as long as Zika was spreading in Puerto Rico and other places where U.S. travelers frequented. When these travelers brought Zika back to neighborhoods where the Aedes aegypti mosquito still lived, sporadic outbreaks could continue to result. The risks to pregnant women, however, were small but real—studies showed that microcephaly occurred in the fetus in up to 13 percent of cases—and pregnant women and women of child bearing years continued to be tested in the event of possible exposure from April 2016 onward.

In terms of controlling the mosquito population, Naled was highly effective, and genetically modified mosquitoes were becoming a tool in the fight against disease-carrying mosquitos (and could be used to attempt to eradicate them entirely). In fact, trials of these engineered mosquitoes reduced the local Aedes aegypti populations by 90 percent in the Cayman Islands and reduced Dengue outbreaks by over 90 percent when tried in

Brazil. (non-biting male mosquitoes which breed and create offspring, which die before they can breed.) However, some ethical considerations and unpredictability in terms of outcome soon emerged. Meanwhile, the Zika vaccines have continued through National Institutes of Health–guided human trials.

PART TWO

COVID

WHAT WE DON'T KNOW DOES HURT US: CHINA AND THE W.H.O.

Back in January, 2020, a novel coronavirus erupted in the central region of China, infecting well over 100,000 people, likely double or triple or even ten times that, killing many thousands, most of them living in the city of Wuhan, a city with a population of more than 11 million people. Like the 2003 Severe Acute Respiratory Syndrome, which had infected over 8,000 and killed close to 800, this new coronavirus came from bats, but what happened after that? Did it species jump to another exotic mammal, perhaps the scaly ugly curved-back pangolin, and then mutate again to a form where it could be transmitted easily from human to human? Coronaviruses were harbored in mammals, and people in this area of China lived closely with their animals, regularly visited bat caves, and some also ate exotic mammals—including bats and pangolins—uncooked as delicacies. This unhealthy practice helped spread the fear of the new Wuhan coronavirus. A video of an unidentified woman eating a quivering bat carcass went viral on social media in late January. Bats were notorious for harboring multiple viruses including nipah, rabies, and coronaviruses, which, when they adapted to humans and spread among us readily, were particularly dangerous and deadly.

But was this the real story? Speculation and conspiracy theories soon abounded throughout the Internet and social media. Was the new contagion bioengineered? Could it be a simple coincidence that the top secret Wuhan virology facility was close by? Had this been a lab accident or a deliberate action by the Politburo of the Communist party? Serious scientists presented their doomsday theories on Youtube, seemingly oblivious to the idea that an engineered bioweapon would not only be more deadly than this one, but would also be identifiable to scientists studying it intensely via an electronmicroscope and biochemical immunoassays. Genetic editors, including CRISPR CAS-9, left a signature.

But even when Chinese scientists published the viral sequence online, and scientist after scientist around the world asserted that there was no sign of genetic manipulation or bioengineering, it did little to silence the conspiracy theorists. The Journal of Medical Virology published a paper which reported that the viral sequence was 88 percent consistent with a bat virus, (SARS had originated with bats as well, before spreading to civet cats and on to humans). But the paper also revealed that the structure included snake genetic sequences as well, specifically either the many-banded krait, or the Chinese cobra. Though a coronavirus had never been associated with reptiles before, fear of snakes spread rapidly around the globe and people began to hunt and kill them, until another scientist debunked this theory and it was replaced by the hideous scaly mammal pangolin as the supposed intermediary mammal. Pangolin scales were traded on the black market and the animal was consumed as exotic food with supposed medicinal value. The pangolin as a cause of this contagion frightened as many people as bats or snakes did.

As public fear ramped up, the American public ricocheted from one theory to another. Just when people had settled on the pangolin theory, learning and espousing the theory of "zoonotic spillover," where an animal virus spreads among humans by continued frequent contact, more conspiracy theories centering on the Wuhan Virology Lab surfaced in the media. It turned out that our National Institutes of Health had been funding research there for several years, for the stated purpose of helping the lab keep up to universal safety standards. Scientists from the NIH insisted that it was far less likely that one of the bat coronaviruses under study would jump to a human scientist or technician than for it to happen in a bat cave or a wet market, where the animal to human contact was much greater. An increasingly anxious public struggled to believe this, and the conspiracy theories died down again, but then further information leaked from a State Department memo that the NIH was actually funding "Gain of Function" research, where a virus is deliberately manipulated or studied to test its ability to mutate to a form where it can jump to and spread among humans. NIH scientists argued that knowing the potential for viral transmission is a good way to be prepared against a possible bioweapon rather than a way to actually create one. But this argument had little traction, the public was slow to understand the semantics here, fear and uncertainty were rampant, obscuring the far greater likelihood of a wet market or bat cave origin, and the conspiracy theories flourished anew.

IN LATE JANUARY, I first covered the story about a deadly coronavirus emerging in China and I tweeted out that any problem for a country as big as China, with 1.5 billion people, was a problem for the world. There was no such thing as a regional infectious health issue in China. But you couldn't tell the extent of this by the response of the World Health Organization (WHO), led by Tedros Adhanom, a public health official and the first non-physician to run the organization.

From a fear point of view, nothing is worse than feeling out of control and playing catch up with a killer virus.

One problem was that China would not let the U.S. bring CDC officers in to monitor and examine the situation. Another problem was that though Dr. Anthony Fauci (head of the National Institute of Allergy and Infectious Disease) and Dr. Robert Redfield (head of the CDC) both told me they had good relationships with the Chinese scientists and that the structure of the virus itself was published online for scientists everywhere to learn from, at the same time, the emerging coronavirus ended up being far more contagious, and caused far more damage to the body in particularly susceptible individuals than we were ever led to believe by China or the WHO. This coronavirus induced damage including: lung inflammation from a hyperimmune response known as cytokine storm, multi-organ inflammation involving the inside lining of blood vessels (endothelium), and blood clotting. All we learned from China was about fever, cough, shortness of breath, and a 15 percent potential for serious pneumonia. We were completely unprepared for this virus, and learned everything as it was happening to us, the same as Europe. This lack of foreknowledge amidst a viral onslaught bred enormous fear.

In fact, it was the job of the WHO to inform and warn the world, which was one of the reasons I backed the president's decision (on Tucker Carlson Tonight) to cut off funding to the WHO and not to restore it after their deeply disturbing failures to inform the world. More than that, it was clear to me that Tedros and his deputy director in charge of communicable diseases, Dr. Ren, who had been a public health official in China for 30 years, were in fact pandering to the Chinese Politburo.

Check out this timeline:

January 14: Tweet from WHO citing Chinese health officials who claimed there had been no human transmissions of the novel coronavirus within the country yet.

January 21: According to German intelligence sources, per the newspaper Der Spiegel, Director Tedros received a call from Chairman Xi of China urging him to delay warning the world and to conceal evidence of person-to-person transmission of the novel coronavirus.

January 23: WHO Director General Tedros issued a statement that the novel coronavirus was a regional problem only.

January 28: After meeting with Chairman Xi, Tedros gushed that "it is admirable that the Chinese government has shown its solid political resolve and taken timely and effective measures in dealing with the epidemic."

January 30: Tedros said, "the Chinese government is to be congratulated for the extraordinary measures it has taken. I left in absolutely no doubt about China's commitment to transparency." Tedros added that they had set "a new standard for outbreak response."

February 3: After visiting Beijing, Tedros continued to praise Chairman Xi's commitment to stopping this outbreak. He also said it was okay to go on with international travel and trade (President Trump was restricting travel from China since **January 31**) Meanwhile, Chairman Xi was banning internal travel from Wuhan, yet allowing international travel to Europe where the coronavirus quickly spread.

February 7: Dr. Li Wenliang, age 34, opthalmologist in Wuhan, died of coronavirus. Warning in a chat room post on December 30th of the new virus, saying it resembled Severe Acute Respiratory Syndrome (SARS), he was visited by the police and forced to sign a statement denouncing his warning as an unfounded and illegal rumor.

February 10: Tedros, "But for now, it's only a spark."

February 15: Munich securities conference: Tedros, China's attempt to control this outbreak has "bought the world time."

March 7: The WHO was still not calling it a pandemic—Public health officials in the U.S., including me, were already calling it a pandemic.

March 11: WHO finally called it a pandemic. A University of Southampton study suggested that China could have reduced the number of coronavirus cases by 95 percent had they moved to contain it just three weeks earlier.

May 14: Dr. Ren Minghui, Assistant Director-General of the WHO in charge of Communicable Diseases, had been a public health official in China for 30 years—tweeted that the "COVID-19 pandemic is highlighting the need to urgently increase services for #MentalHealth or risk a massive increase in mental health conditions in the coming months."

I responded on *Tucker Carlson Tonight* on Fox News that though I completely agreed with this sentiment, on the other hand, had the WHO done what they were supposed to do and warned us rather than aiding and abetting the spread of the virus around the world, perhaps we wouldn't be in such mental health trouble with enormous damage to the world's psyche.

THE QUARANTINE CENTER IN MID AMERICA

In late February, people in the U.S. were not yet afraid. They should have been. I travelled with my producer and crew for *Tucker Carlson Tonight* to the National Quarantine Center at Nebraska Medicine, where we were able to determine through unprecedented access to the teams nurses and doctors that the novel coronavirus was easily transmissible and had already likely spread throughout many communities in the U.S. The center was treating 15 patients from the Diamond Princess Cruise Ship off the coast of Japan. 13 of the 15 had tested positive and two were in the more intensive biocontainment unit, suffering from pneumonia. One of these patients was receiving the anti-viral drug remdesivir, which at the time was just beginning to be studied for this virus, under the direction of Dr. Andre Kalil, who I interviewed. The medical professionals treating these patients were heroes, caring for the patients while at the same time studying the coronavirus closely. They were making extremely useful determinations that no one else had before made.

The conditions in the quarantine rooms were good. Jeri Seratti-Goldman, one of the patients who had not tested positive for the coronavirus (her husband Carl was in biocontainment), told us that the food was good and she benefited from sticking to the same daily routine that she follows at home. She worked out on a treadmill and then works on her computer.

"Keeping busy has helped my psyche quite a bit," Seratti-Goldman said. "Keeping a positive attitude and knowing that this is all out of our control, so I just have to roll."

"I was not frightened until yesterday," she said, "my good friends from St. George, Utah, Mark and Jerri Jorgenson. Jerri was the first to contract the virus. Mark was diagnosed and he got a positive yesterday. I guess this is the first time I've been frightened. In my head I was hoping that tomorrow was day ten. . . . Bummed that he tested positive and there is still a possibility for me to test positive."

"Three people a day come in at breakfast, lunch and dinner, they give you your meals and check your temperature," Seratti-Goldman continued. "And that's the only contact I have." She suffered a broken tooth and the staff had to go out and get her some Bondo (putty glue) because there was no way to have anyone come in and fix it.

Dr. Jeffrey Gold, chancellor at the University of Nebraska Medical Center, was the first to indicate in an interview with us that the virus appeared to be far more contagious than the flu, and therefore would be very difficult to contain. Gold said he was looking to the response in countries like South Korea, Japan and Italy, which had much better-developed health care infrastructures than China's, to predict whether the novel coronavirus would evade travel restrictions and take route in the U.S. He was not alone. Many experts in late February and early March were hoping that our advanced health care system could contain this virus, and of course, this turned out not to be the case.

Kate Boulter, lead nurse for the biocontainment unit, and nurse Grant Fabry met with us in the biocontainment unit "brain room" and demonstrated how personal protective equipment worked. They pointed out that they are being extra cautious at the University of Nebraska Medical Center, but the basic uniform of disposable N95 respirator mask, gown, gloves and face shield should be sufficient. This ended up being the "uniform" that health care workers encountering patients with the coronavirus donned throughout the Spring and Summer. The team at Nebraska helped disrobe each other after each encounter so no virus can possibly be spread. The buddy system, too, was adopted around the country in the months to come.

Nurse Shelly Schwedhelm, the highly skilled director of the National Center for Health Security and Biopreparedness at the University of Nebraska Medical Center, told us that in terms of preparedness for COVID-19, "there's a long way to go." This ended up being a hauntingly prophetic comment, as did the statement from Acting Deputy Secretary of Homeland Security, Ken Cuccinelli, who I had interviewed at Dulles Airport right before flying to Nebraska. He said, "Our borders are no guarantee that the virus won't find its way here . . . really, what we are trying to do is slow down the virus getting here and reduce the impact when it does get here. (We are dealing with) first world countries that have outstanding health care systems and yet the speed of virus spread is very high."

During my live appearances in the frigid cold from outside the Nebraska Medicine Global Center for Health Security, I interviewed Nurse Schwedhelm live, and threw to the tape of my interview with Cuccinelli. In that tape I warned the world in my own words too, but I suppose it was hard for viewers at the time, back in February, to conceptualize how severe this risk actually was, "the virus is slipping into the United States," I said. "We still have very few coronavirus test kits around, so we don't know how much of the virus there is, and we also still don't know how contagious it is, and we don't know how deadly it is. But one thing we do know, people are continuing to come to the United States, many of whom are travelling from countries where the coronavirus is spreading."

As Sarah Connor said so famously in the movie *The Terminator*, a storm was coming.

UP ON THE COVID RECOVERY WARDS

The last weekend in April, on the COVID-19 wards at NYU Langone Orthopedic Hospital, it was the new business as usual. Namely, helping patients wean off oxygen, treating their anxiety and blood clots in their legs, and overcoming fatigue and deconditioning. I participated and learned a lot about the twists and turns of recovery. The virus and its aftermath could ravage the body, badly damaging the lungs, heart, kidneys, and brain. Rehabilitation was difficult, not to mention the problems of when and where to send the patients when they were medically ready to leave.

Were two negative tests for COVID-19 sufficient before someone could go back to a household with an elderly parent or immuno-compromised spouse? Where should a homeless patient go? These were the questions of the day. Treating this disease was a long slow process that didn't end at the hospital door.

At the heart of the battle in New York City was NYU Langone Health. Its orthopedic hospital took COVID transfers from Tisch Hospital and the Kimmel Pavillion, NYU Winthrop and NYU Brooklyn while at the same time, according to the chair of orthopedic surgery, Dr. Joseph Zuckerman, also accepting transfers for orthopedic emergencies from Bellevue, Tisch and other hospitals that were beset by COVID patients.

Langone Orthopedic Hospital itself had four COVID wards filled with patients in various stages of recovery. The hospital had temporarily pivoted and changed its overall purpose to perform as a transition hospital for COVID-19 patients. According to Nurse Practitioner AB Brody, just coming off an overnight shift, there was an unsettling amount of unpredictability to the virus. He described to me the plight of a 93-year-old woman who had multiple medical problems, and was turning blue with very low oxygen levels in the middle of the night. They turned her over (proning) and she stabilized, the team gave her extra oxygen, which she responded to, and within four days she turned everything around in a positive direction and was able to go home. Brody added, sadly, that there were other patients, including some younger ones, who had not done nearly as well, and some had died.

Dr. James Slover, in charge of the surgical service at the hospital, talked to me about how the teams had come together, sharing skills, a hospitalist, nurse practitioner and physicians assistants working together with the orthopedists who usually inhabited these halls. Slover indicated that they were all learning from each other, that a surgical nurse practitioner with expertise in Personal Protective Equipment quickly shared this information, while at the same time learning standard medical practices from his or her medical cohorts.

Michelle Meneses, Manager of Advanced Practice Providers at the hospital, but now managing COVID Medicine, talked to me about the challenges of treating both mental and physical disabilities in COVID patient recovery. The anxiety that stemmed from this illness, the isolation and the fear, compounded pre-existing psychiatric conditions and made adjustment and placement that much harder.

Recovery from COVID-19 was a long game. It required not just retooling but constant commitment and devotion. As I walked through the wards clothed in PPR, I couldn't get out of my head the image of Dr. Adam Karp, a highly regarded longtime geriatrician, clearly in a high risk group because of his weight and being over 60 years old, carefully donned PPE to enter the room of a recovering COVID patient, bringing good cheer while performing an important decanulation procedure—removing the breathing tube from the patient's trachea—a high exposure event for Karp which demonstrated that the patient was on the road to recovery.

Dr. Karp did not appear afraid and then I saw why. He was wearing a kippah on the back of his head, and I didn't have to ask him to know that he was on the wards to do God's work. He and everyone else there appeared unafraid and performed their assignments at a high level. It was all about courage and caring to overcome fear. This jewel of a hospital would not be defeated by this powerful virus.

SCIENCE VERSUS THE POLITICS OF COVID

Back in mid March, my father, who was 96 years old, felt suddenly fatigued, with some shortness of breath and fever. He lay down on his couch and said he didn't think he was ever going to get up again. He has heart disease and a pacemaker, and his cardiologist weighed the options and agreed to start him on hydroxychloroquine and zithromax. He was much better within a day. I made the same decision in several patients with COVID, or suspected COVID, in my practice over the first few months of the pandemic, prescreening them for risk of heart rhythm abnormalities. I understood that the benefits I saw were anecdotal, and not strictly scientific.

Still, I was glad when the U.S. Food and Drug Administration issued an Emergency Use Authorization (EUA) for hospital use on March 28th. A study around the same time in *Nature* demonstrated hydroxychloroquine's anti-viral activity against the SARS COV 2 virus that is responsible for COVID-19. There was also longtime evidence that the drug decreased inflammation that could lead to the "cytokine storm" that damages the lungs in severely ill COVID patients. There was every reason to be excited. The drug was incredibly cheap, a generic version was less than 50 cents per pill, and it has been around for more than 65 years. It had been well tolerated by millions as a treatment for various forms of arthritis and as a preventative against malaria. On top of its medical value, there was the usefulness of a drug you could rely on as a reassurance against the fear of being exposed to COVID or against the need for hospitalization if the symptoms became severe.

But then the bad news began to pour in. With President Trump championing the drug in early April, it became a third rail political issue, and studies (including one from New York published in the *Journal of the American Medical Association* in May) showed that the drug wasn't effective against COVID, at least very late in the game when the patient was dying, and side effects of the drug were also more likely at that point. The political fallout interfered with the science. Soon after President Trump admitted to taking it as a prophylactic on May 25th, the FDA revoked its EUA on June 15th. Another study from Oxford University published in *Lancet* showed the drug to be ineffective when given to very sick patients, and even to hasten death. But the study was soon withdrawn because of relying on faulty data from a questionable company, Surgisphere, with few employees and unverified data.

Instead of learning a lesson from the failed *Lancet* study, that more carefully conducted research was essential, especially early in the disease or as a preventative, the NIH and the WHO both stopped their clinical trials on hydroxychloroquine. It was the politics of fear all over again.

Luckily, one bold and innovative group did not stop. In early July, the Henry Ford Health System in Detroit released a large retrospective study where the drug was given very early in the hospitalization. I spoke with the Chief Academic Officer there, neurosurgeon Dr. Steve Kalkanis, who said, "We stand behind our recent Henry Ford study where we looked at 2,500 patients and we found that the use of hydroxychloroquine alone cut the death rate in half (from 26 percent to 13 percent)." According to Kalkanis, the study screened heavily for those with pre-existing conditions including cardiac disease. He believed that the key to success was using the drug early in the course of the illness, before significant inflammation occurs.

In mid July a placebo double-blind randomized study released by the University of Minnesota published in the *Annals of Internal Medicine* showed that hydroxychloroquine did not work to decrease symptoms in mild to moderate cases among outpatients. I had interviewed one of the study's lead authors, Dr. Sarah Lofgren, on Doctor Radio, and appeared with her on TV, and I believed that she had every expectation the study would turn out positive. This led me to be more swayed by a negative result, and to say so on Fox News, but afterward, I found out that the study, which utilized online volunteers, did not confirm whether they were actually diagnosed with COVID or not, but went by symptoms alone, weakening their analysis. We were still looking for the gold standard of medical research, a double-blinded prospective randomized trial, and also in July, a randomized study from Brazil published in the *New England Journal of Medicine* showed no effect against COVID-19 in mild to moderate hospitalized patients. This might have put the controversy to bed, but critics pointed out that the study enrolled people on average 7 days into their hospitalization, far too late to conclude that the treatment didn't work early on or as an outpatient.

Also in July, Congressman Dr. Michael Burgess of Texas, Republican leader on the House Subcommittee on Health, told me that he was receiving calls from all over the country asking why the drug wasn't in front line use. He said that doctors in Texas he spoke to were now afraid to prescribe it because the FDA, led by Dr. Stephen Hahn, had withdrawn the Emergency Use Authorization, which, though it didn't apply directly to outpatient off label (without specific FDA indication) use, still set a precedent that Burgess felt left doctors open to lawsuits if anything went wrong.

The original purpose of the EUA on hydroxychloroquine was to get access to a stockpile in Pakistan (Bayer). Unfortunately, according to a senior administration official I spoke to in August, the FDA had "screwed up" and applied it to across-the-board hospital use. It was really never needed, and withdrawing it sent the wrong message. There was already plenty of the drug around, including 50 million doses from Teva. The amount from Bayer was much less.

The drug needed to be given at the right point in the process. Sadly, the jury was still out on this. For the most part, the drug was tested far too late when patients were already too sick for its potential anti-viral or anti-inflammatory effects to work.

When I spoke with Dr. Hahn on Doctor Radio on SiriusXM, he indicated that several studies on use of hydroxychloroquine early in the course of COVID-19 were still ongoing, and he echoed that the only reason FDA had withdrawn the EUA was because supplies to hospitals were plentiful. But the impact of this move backfired, as the president's economic advisor Peter Navarro indicated to me when he backed a group of Henry Ford doctors who unsuccessfully lobbied the FDA to reinstitute the EUA.

Unfortunately, this entire battle was about politics rather than medicine. The end result was to make the public more afraid, one group (mostly on the right politically) championed hydroxychloroquine and advocated its use, even as it became restricted in more states and more pharmacies across the country. The political left, on the other hand, denounced the drug based on flawed science and continued to ridicule President Trump for having used it himself.

Meanwhile, the science crept along. The Henry Ford group was also studying the drug as a preventive in 3000 health care workers and there was an ongoing study at my medical center, NYU Langone Health, which was looking at the combination of hydroxychloroquine and zinc to prevent or treat COVID-19 early in the course of the disease.

And then, in early August, the ultimate tie breaker seemed to appear. A randomized prospective double-blinded trial was published in the *New England Journal of Medicine* of more than 800 people concluded that hydroxychloroquine, when given to people who had had significant exposure to the coronavirus were not less likely to develop the illness and were in fact more likely to have side effects—from the drug. But then it turned out that this was the same group at Minnesota. The trial methods did not allow consistent proof of exposure to SARS-CoV-2 or consistent laboratory confirmation that the symptom complex that was reported represented a SARS-CoV-2 infection. Also, the mean age of participants was 40, so by age alone they were less likely to experience a severe case of COVID.

"So, what are we to do with the results of this trial? The advocacy and widespread use of hydroxychloroquine seem to reflect a reasonable fear of SARS-CoV-2 infection. However, it would appear that to some extent the media and social forces—rather than medical evidence—are driving clinical decisions and the global COVID-19 research agenda," said Myron S. Cohen MD, Director, Institute for Global Health & Infectious Diseases, University of North Carolina at Chapel Hill, Chapel Hill.

I couldn't have said it better myself. I continued to hope the FDA and the NIH would reverse their course and continue to participate in clinical trials for early and prophylactic use of the drug. I began to wonder if the lack of motivation wasn't more tied to economics than science, as Navarro suggested.

I couldn't say for certain that my father and several of my patients survived COVID because of hydroxychloroquine, but I wanted science to prove me wrong, not politics. We desperately needed treatments for COVID-19, not dogma and divisiveness.

A treatment or vaccine made you feel better protected against an unseen viral killer, much as a fortified entrance or a guard dog caused you to feel protected against a prowler. Knowing that the anti-viral drug remdesivir and the steroid dexamethasone had emerged as effective in-hospital treatments for COVID was of some comfort, but people across the country wanted to know what they might take as a preventative, or for early treatment in case they got sick. This was especially important as we waited for a vaccine to emerge, hopefully by the beginning of 2021.

Convalescent antibodies (taken from recovering patients) had provided early treatment for many conditions, dating back to the late 19th century. They had been useful before vaccines became available for diptheria, polio, measles, and hepatitis B. Nowadays we also had the option of targeted synthetic antibodies, which were generally more potent and more effective and they were being studied for use against the SARS-CoV-2 virus that causes COVID-19.

In August, Mayo Clinic released promising results of a study on convalescent plasma, also known as passive immunity, where antibodies from a recovering patient were introduced to help those most ill. Overall, 70,000 people were studied, with 35,000 of these overseen by Mayo. They weren't strictly randomized, but some got high dose and some got low dose plasma, and some received none, which was a good measure. At 7 days and at 30 days the survival rate was better for those who got the treatment, more so with the higher amount. And yet, the FDA first dragged its feet at issuing an Emergency Use Authorization, despite the fact that this was not the same thing as fully licensing a drug. The fact was, it has been used for 116 years successfully for other diseases, and it was clear that it had an affect on very sick patients with COVID, and should be utilized, especially right in the middle of a pandemic. The EUA should have been automatic. Politics, coming out of the NIH, supervened.

Another promising treatment under investigation was the inhaled steroid ciclesonide, which had been found to have anti-viral properties against this coronavirus and also acted as an anti-inflammatory agent. Pulmonologists already used it all the time to treat asthma and allergic rhinitis. The drug's effectiveness against COVID-19 was largely anecdotal, but clinical trials were ongoing.

I didn't understand why most of the studies on hydroxychloroquine involved hospitalized patients, because by the time patients were really sick or in the ICU, they were frequently suffering from lung and other organ inflammation and blood clotting problems.

There was no reason to believe that hydroxychloroquine would work at this point, and multiple studies had confirmed the ineffectiveness of the drug. Its potential side effects in terms of cardiac arrhythmias had long been known, as the drug has been on the market (as prophylaxis against malaria and treatment for lupus) for over sixty years.

And by the middle of August, considering hydroxychloroquine as a preventive or early treatment for COVID-19 appeared to be almost over except among heretics or outliers. Its use has been tainted, not just by negative research and by the FDA withdrawing its Emergency Use Authorization (which has made doctors afraid to prescribe it for fear of lawsuits), but by the politicization of the drug over President Trump's endorsement and subsequent admission that he was taking it.

Back in March, things were different. A study out of China had showed the effectiveness of hydroxychloroquine as an anti-viral agent against this coronavirus and there was every reason to study it further. A top pulmonologist I worked with took it when he got COVID, and he was not alone.

He felt better, but didn't know if it was the drug or not. My father, who is in his mid 90's, felt very fatigued one day, had a fever and chest pain, and said he didn't think he could get up from the couch. His cardiologist prescribed hydroxychloroquine and azithromycin and by the next day, he felt much better.

It was hard for me to believe it wasn't the treatment working, in fact, it is still hard for me to believe it, though I realize now that we were probably treating our fear of the virus as much as of the virus itself. Perhaps I would still like to see the well conducted large double-blinded placebo controlled randomized trial—for early use—that has yet to be done. And many experts including scientists at NYU believe that zinc is the crucial ingredient needed to get hydroxychloroquine to work.

And consider this. the word anecdote may be used too dismissively. The fact was, my father was 96 years old, and a tough World War II veteran who was not prone to exaggeration. He also had multiple medical problems including a recent heart valve replacement, and at his age didn't have much reserve left. when he said he felt he was a "goner," there was no reason not to believe him. his recovery after taking hydroxychloroquine was dramatic, which was still not proof of course, but it certainly gave me pause when we tested his COVID antibodies several weeks later and they came back positive.

Back in March, we had nothing else to offer. By August we were much more inclined to wait patiently for the scientific proof to back up our choices, even though, as the virus continued to spread, the tendency to follow our intuition recurred.

LOCKDOWNS AND THE
POLITICS OF FEAR

In early August I travelled to Atlanta to fill in for Dr. Mehmet Oz at a below-the-radar conference of doctors/entrepreneurs. It was a quick turn around trip and I was back on Long Island the same evening. Oz ended up appearing remotely and we were a great tag team, as I socially distanced, wearing a clear mask, on a stage far away from my audience, and talked about overcoming fears and never giving up. I told stories about my mountain bike rides with former President Bush and my recent interview with President Trump; when he'd invited me to join him in the Oval Office and I said that I was brought up in Queens too, a few miles from him, and that I was a fighter too.

"You are a fighter," he said, acknowledging that I had received my share of unfair media attacks.

"Where in Queens do you live now?"

"Not in Queens. I have a house on the water in Sag Harbor."

"Whoo hoo hoo," he said, grinning, and I laughed, knowing that he could buy my whole street in a minute. I was flown in and flown out, so although Atlanta was a current hot spot, I wasn't subject to a quarantine on returning to New York. This was a disturbing corollary to the COVID leadership inconsistencies that had riddled Governor Cuomo from the beginning of the pandemic, which I refer to in the chapter on fear leaders. Nursing homes had responded to a state directive and had readmitted COVID-19 patients even though they did not have proper facilities and staffing to handle them, and nursing home patients were, of course, very susceptible to the ravages of COVID. It spread there easily and more than 6,000 patients died.

I had to wonder if this arbitrary 24 hour window which, allowed me to fly in and out of New York without quarantine, wasn't deliberately added to the statute in order to help high level business executives. It certainly made no sense when it came to public health, when I considered that 24 hours was more than enough time to catch or transmit a coronavirus. It also made the news when people were able to fly from overseas for the MTV video awards without being fully quarantined.

Still, I had to admit that Governor Cuomo and his health commissioner Dr. Howard Zucker had done an excellent job overall at setting a standard for public health compliance including social distancing, masking, bar and restaurant and gym closures, and later, restrictions that had no doubt contributed in a major way to the significant drop off in cases. New York, which had been among the worst cities hit with COVID, now had less than 700 new cases per day and a rate positivity percentage of less than one percent.

My parents, in their mid nineties, had flown back to New York from Florida—a hot spot—in early July, had been subject to the quarantine, and my father had actually received a call from a New York State health department official every day for two weeks to make sure he was at home.

At the conference I picked up a pin with a red slash through the statement "No Hugging" instead of "No smoking." I thought it was a white badge, like the no smoking signs of yore, but when I took it out of my travel bag to show on TV the following night, it turned out to be yellow. Still, it looked enough like the "no smoking" pin that I showed it on TV and suggested that we use it in schools (along with "no hugging" shirts), at least until a vaccine appeared. Tucker Carlson said he couldn't go along with it completely, as he was a hugger, which I said I was too. Still, I felt that I was conveying a message of restraint that might be useful in schools as a way of staying open. The implied message was that hugging could be a way of spreading the virus if there was already some of it in the schools.

Somehow I tapped into a vein of fear among the COVID deniers, and I was attacked by a group of anti-vaxxers on social media. Many drew a comparison between my yellow pin and the yellow stars that Jewish children were forced to wear as identifiers in the Nazi-run Warsaw ghetto. Several enraged tweeters went so far as to call me, a religious Jew whose great grandparents had been killed in a pogrom, a Nazi, or Dr. Mengele. I was deeply hurt, and reported several of these tweets and blocked the sender, but it took several days for the assault on my sensibility and identity to stop.

I finally concluded that the anger and rage against me came from the place of frustration and fear that so many were feeling, blurring boundaries. Still, it was inexcusable. No Jew should ever be called a Nazi.

I was reminded of something I had said on Tucker's show two weeks before, when I was responding to the question of why I had let the president give full answers during my interview and had not interrupted him. I said that I wasn't brought up to interrupt people, that I considered it a sign of respect. Tucker added (interrupting me for the first time ever on the show), that it was also because the whole purpose of an interview was to learn what the other person has to say, not to hear myself speak, and I had done that.

"Kindness and respect," I said to Tucker's audience of millions, was my prescription for the weekend. "Respect and kindness."

Kindness and empathy are emotions that flow through the same centers of the brain as fear. They are an antidote.

IN MODERN TIMES, lockdowns first occurred in 1918, during the Spanish Flu pandemic that killed 675,000 people in the U.S. and over 50 million people around the world. I have discussed this with several experts, including Dr. Anthony Fauci, and I believe this model has led, in part, to the lockdowns we have been experiencing now, beginning with Wuhan, China, and on to Italy, France, Spain, and several states here in the U.S.

New Zealand and Australia are different, because they are island countries where complete travel bans are more easily accomplished, and in fact, New Zealand successfully locked down with more than one hundred days in the middle of the pandemic without a single new case.

But travel bans are the key, and they are very difficult to enact in regions where plane travel is still going on and in the case of COVID-19, may be dishonest about their symptoms, their point of origin, or simply taken Tylenol to suppress a fever.

Back in 1918, Health Commissioner Dr. Max Starkloff learned that the Spanish Flu was resurging in Boston in the Fall (second wave), and he prevailed on Mayor Henry Kiel to allow him to shut down most of St. Louis on October 7th, three days after the first reported case of influenza in the city, leading to fewer cases, hospitalizations, and deaths, at least initially. You may find all of this familiar—bars and indoor dining at restaurants suspended, bowling alleys and gyms, churches, dance halls, theaters, and barbershops shuttered, schools and most places of business closed, even most funerals. Travel on street cars was restricted, but of course there were no airplanes. Starkloff believed in "social distancing," and the death rate in St. Louis was 2.8 per 1,000 residents, lowest among the nation's major cities, compared to 8 in Pittsburgh, and 7.6 in San Francisco.

The key to his success was early action, *before* the contagion had taken hold.

Flash forward to 2020 and COVID. It was not the lack of an across-the-board lockdown that enabled COVID-19 to spread throughout the country, it was the lack of consistent compliance to public health measures intended to control spread. Keep in mind that by the time lockdowns were instituted in the U.S. in March, the SARS COV 2 virus had already spread throughout our communities. I was warned of this back in late February, when I travelled to the Nebraska Medical Center National Quarantine Unit, and I was told of the imperfect system of detection at Dulles Airport by more than one Custom and Border Protection agent. Travelers didn't always admit they originated in China or that they weren't feeling well.

Lockdowns, in order to be most effective, must occur before a highly transmissible virus is deeply embedded, and they must be accompanied by complete travel shutoff to and from hot spots, as was the case in New Zealand, and to some extent, in Australia. Neither was the case here.

In fact, an inadequate public health response on the part of both our private and public health care system including our Centers for Disease Control and Prevention (which delayed important testing and identification of cases for weeks) helped spread both fear and virus. We all expected more of our resources, our technology, and our manpower. Instead, we were not alerted to how pervasive the problem was until our hospitals were flooded in New York and our precious health care workers put at risk.

But instead of a laser surgical approach to our emerging hot spots (New York and New Jersey at first and later Florida, Texas, Arizona, and California), panic ensued, and most of the country shut down, including rural states with few cases such as Montana, Wyoming, and Maine. Economies were strangled, millions of jobs were lost, medical care of all kinds was delayed, and depression and anxiety soared. South Dakota resisted, and did not show a peak in cases as a result. In fact, as of August 7th, 2020, there were still less than 10,000 COVID cases in the entire state. Unfortunately, too few have paid attention to South Dakota's contrary example.

The essential public health problem was never about shutting down one region more than another, it was about compliance variations within hot spot communities, leading to more viral spread, eventually to high risk groups, overwhelming hospitals. Whereas some of us were hunkered down, wearing masks, washing hands and physically distancing, others were out cavorting at bars or restaurants (when open) with their masks hanging off their faces, shouting and drinking.

The more non-compliant one half of Americans were, the more pressure there was on the rest of us to police ourselves or be policed. It became a political problem, with the Democrats becoming the party of extreme lockdowns, schools closing, universal masking, wide expansive testing, roadblocks to emerging drugs—the party of fear in this case, whereas the Republicans were the party of reopening, the party of innovation, of throwing research caution to the wind for old and new treatments, the party of schools staying open and testing only those who were symptomatic and surveilling the rest, looking for hot spots.

These were the same problems that communities and cities faced during the 1918 Spanish Flu pandemic. It often felt like we hadn't learned anything about public health since then. Yesteryear's draft rallies and parades, which spread the dreaded flu during WWI, were today's protests and large gatherings.

I could see that we could be living in a science fiction world soon; as someone over the age of 60, I could soon be wearing a Hazmat suit with a PAPPR rebreathing unit standing across the street from a shouting maskless person at a demonstration.

When it comes to public health, exemptions from a deadly virus were not excusable. Of course, if we didn't fully test or contact trace people at a protest, we couldn't prove that people were transmitting the virus there, even if the protest or riot took place in a hot spot.

I believed that from the beginning of the pandemic, we needed to focus more on emerging hotspots rather than on shutting down the whole country. Though outbreaks in the west (and prior to this in the South) had a higher percentage of younger patients with milder cases, still, in all places the virus spread eventually to the elderly, the obese, and those most at risk and the hospitals and ICUs filled. Sources on the ground in Florida, California, and Texas told me in June and July they were dealing with a similar situation as we had here in New York.

MY MOTHER WAS out on the front porch, sitting in a beach lounge chair from the 1960s, that I barely remembered from my early childhood and hadn't seen since. I was so glad to see her, she and my father had just returned from Florida, where they had been sequestered in their retirement community as the virus raged around them. They are both in their mid nineties, and now that they were back in their Long Island house they were subject to a two week quarantine under the orders of Governor Cuomo. In fact, government health officials were calling every single day to check on their whereabouts. New York was doing well when it came to COVID-19, and so were my parents.

Hospitals were back to almost normal function, which meant that cancer screenings and important surgeries were ongoing. It is easy to call a procedure elective unless it is your hernia, or your gallbladder, or your cardiac stent we are talking about. My own hospital, NYU Langone, was fully up and running, and I was back in the office, seeing patients, albeit with a mask and shield.

I am not sure what prompted the story, since I wasn't talking about hospitals on my parent's porch, unless my mother was reading my mind as mothers often do.

"My brother had to go into the hospital in 1918 only there was no room," she said.

"Your brother. This was before you were born. He was seven years older than you. What was his name?"

She hesitated. "Leonard. His name was Leonard. After what happened, my mother didn't want to have any more children. It took her seven years to change her mind."

My mother seemed sad with the memory. Leonard. My uncle Leonard.

"He was nine months old."

"Right. You remember. He had an ear infection," she said, pointing to her right ear. "They wanted to take him to the hospital, but all the hospitals were full."

"With the Spanish flu," I said. "Filled with victims of the Spanish Flu."

"That's right. They couldn't get him in and he died."

It was strange to be comforting my mother about something that had happened so long ago.

"There were no antibiotics back then," I said. "Not even sulfa. He would have died anyway. Ear infections went to the brain."

"They wanted to do an operation," she said, pointing to just below her ears."

"Oh, a bilateral mastoidectomy. Right. That could have saved him."
My mother grew teary, and suddenly we both saw the parallel between back then and now. More than a hundred years later, patients in COVID hot spots were not getting the urgent care they needed because the hospitals were already full with a contagious disease or people who needed urgent care were too afraid to go there. With antibiotics taking the place of risky operations, we had the treatments we needed to save lives like poor Uncle Leonard's, but people were afraid and the access to care was shrinking.

Too many things had not changed since 1918. We continued to have gatherings right in the middle of a pandemic. Protests instead of draft rallies, but regardless, the virus spread.

I wished that Uncle Leonard's memory could serve as a warning. In 1918 few knew what a virus was and could predict its impact. But what was our excuse now over a hundred years later?

ONE OF THE few scientists to study the impact of the Spanish Flu on mental health was Norwegian scientist Svenn-Erik Mamelund. He found that the number of first time psychiatric hospitalizations increased by several times following the pandemic in Norway. He also found an increased rate of suicide in the U.S. and mental disturbances among Spanish flu survivors.

The numbers aren't in yet for COVID, but it is clear that the pandemic has had a huge impact on mental health.

THE PRESIDENT:
IN REAL TIME

Americans have come to falsely believe that we can evaluate our leaders based on TV snippets.

Doctors too easily fell into this trap and should not have been diagnosing people they had never met. The American Psychiatric Association's famed Goldwater rule was more applicable now than ever. The rule emanated from *Fact Magazine* publishing a survey of psychiatrists calling Senator (and presidential candidate) Barry Goldwater crazy during the 1964 presidential election.

President Trump has received more than his share of attacks from psychiatrists. Dr. Bandy Lee, a Yale psychiatrist, published a book of essays in late 2017 by numerous mental health experts entitled "The Dangerous Case of Donald Trump." Last December, during the impeachment proceedings, she and others presented a petition to Congress signed by 350 mental health professionals claiming that the president's mental fitness was rapidly declining.

What did these professionals all have in common? They had not met the president.

On July 22nd, 2020, I was invited to the White House to interview President Trump for Fox News. Having never met him before, I spent more than an hour at the interview and in the Oval Office. It was close to 90 degrees outside, but Trump appeared quite comfortable and was not sweating or short of breath. I found him to be nothing at all like he's been described; he was gracious rather than ill-tempered or mean. He was a showman;

choosing the place and camera angles for the interview; standing in the pillared walkway alongside the rose garden.

I was not there to evaluate or provoke him, but rather to ask questions and allow him to answer. This was my brand of journalistic restraint, and it was also how I was brought up to show respect. The interview was about him, not me. He was engaged, focused, displaying empathy, not at all what you would expect of someone with a psychiatric diagnosis. When I asked him about masks, he spoke about his feelings during a recent visit to Walter Reed Military Hospital, "I was seeing young people that were hurt very badly in military situations. And I felt for them, not for me, I felt for them. My wearing a mask was a good thing. I felt extremely comfortable. I don't feel comfortable in other settings when I'm all by myself on a stage and everybody's way far away."

He spoke somberly of the people he'd lost from COVID-19. In the moment, this was not the raging narcissist that Dr. Lee and others have described. "I've lost five people," he said. "Probably six, actually, as of this moment, I think pretty soon. But I've lost five friends that went in. One of them tested—great guy, Stanley Chera, one of the top real estate people in New York, a very successful man, good man who was never into politics until I ran, he became like a political wild man. He loved it, but a great guy with great spirit, he said, I tested positive. And I said, well, that's too bad, but you'll be okay. (He agreed.) I'll be okay. He went to the hospital. Two days later he's in a coma. And two days later he died. And, you know, that's happened on numerous occasions. Probably happened to you with people, too. I never remember anything like that."

This was an interview, not a medical encounter, but in the time I spent with him I saw no evidence of a psychiatric problem being manifested.

With the election coming up, I asked him about candidate health. I said, "presidential health or health of a candidate is going to be on the table, of course, as it always is. And I've been someone always asking for that. And I've seen a lot about you being in good health. What do you think should come out or be the attention regarding Vice President Biden."

He did not attack Biden directly, as he might have done in the past. Talking about himself, he said, ". . . first they'd say he wants to take over the world, he's going to take over the world. He's a dictator. The next day they'll say he's crazy. The next day they'll say, oh, he's incompetent. The next day they'll say . . . something." Trump said he'd had the cognitive test (Montreal

Cognitive Assessment) with Dr. Ronnie Jackson, the former White House physician, in part "to shut these people up there."

Part of the test was remembering five words in order, Trump gave as an example "person, woman, man, camera, TV." Apparently the memory test (Montreal Cognitive Assessment) he'd taken included sequential word memory and he bragged he'd had a very high score. Of course the late night comedians and pundits made a mockery of his grandiosity the way they always do.

But there was more. President Trump was serious about the need for an advanced intellect as a qualification to be president,". . . we have to have somebody that's sharp. Because I can tell you, President Xi is sharp. President Putin is sharp. Erdogan (president of Turkey) is sharp. You don't have any non sharp people that you're dealing with. And we can't have somebody that's not 100 percent." Trump suggested that Biden "should take the test in a way as an obligation too, because you have to be able to show this country that the person that we're picking as leader is sharp . . ."

After the interview, I reached out to the Biden camp, but was unsuccessful in securing an interview.

It was a shame the clip went viral. True it was good TV, great social media, but it also obscured the larger reality of the interview. Trump had shown coherent insights and charisma, traits that could help him to unite us to overcome our fears in a time of terrible crisis, if only more people were receptive, and he could apply these traits consistently.

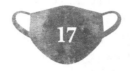

FEAR PROPS:
MASKS

The politics of fear and the power of science. Masks were right in the middle of both. On the science side, there was increasing evidence that masks, when properly used, played a role in decreasing viral spread by, at least, partly blocking respiratory droplets expelled during coughing, sneezing, and even speech. Since there was a buildup of viral particles in the days just before a person became symptomatic, this certainly made sense for COVID. Of course, this was assuming that people wore clean masks that fit their face well, and that they wore them over their noses, not dangling off their chins, and that they didn't wear them instead of physical distancing.

A study published in *Health Affairs* looking at 15 states and Washington D.C. that had mask mandates showed a definite decrease in transmission. Other population studies showed the same, including one among health care workers at Massachusetts General Hospital, and simulations clearly showed that masks (N95 better than surgical, better than cloth) decreased the spread of respiratory droplets. A growing number of observational studies were also revealing that counties and states with mask mandates showed lower case numbers and lower viral transmissions.

Unfortunately, fear attached itself to the situation and masks became a political hot potato, as well as a means to control people. While many were compliant, others rebelled and were deliberately non-compliant.

Former Vice President Joe Biden announced in mid August, as part of his presidential campaign that he was asking for a national mask mandate for all for three months, but he added the word "outside," which raised eyebrows. It was well known that the coronavirus transmitted more easily indoors, in poorly ventilated areas, and if there were to be a national mask mandate, especially intended to target hotspots, it should be razor sharp. President Trump blasted back against the fear mongering, criticizing his opponent for being okay with allowing "rioters and looters and criminals and millions of illegal aliens to roam free in our country." Trump also questioned the science as well, and the authority that a president has to issue such a mandate.

Riding my bicycle around Manhattan, I and everyone else wore masks, which seemed ridiculous, especially since many picnickers around us were rebellious and non-compliant. What was even more absurd was that few bikers wore helmets these days, which to me as a physician meant that there would be far more head injuries than any viral exchange. Such were the effects of fear—it caused an obsession that left out almost everything else. All other public health measures went quickly out the window.

Meanwhile, Harvard researchers were suggesting wearing masks during sex with someone outside your household. The science for that was of course unproven, but the impact on romance was clear, especially if the government were watching.

At the same time, a Wisconsin state agency recommended wearing a mask on a private zoom call even if you were home alone. I recommended no such thing, although I did suggest turning the zoom camera off, in case big brother were in the room.

Masks were one fear prop against COVID—we knew they contributed significantly to helping prevent spread, but we didn't know exactly how much. Definitive double-blinded, randomized studies had never been done. How could they be? How could we subject one maskless group to the virus while another group wore coverings? One study covered a hamster cage with a masklike covering and then blew the virus at them. That group was far less likely to become infected than the maskless group, but this was hardly applicable science.

The confusion and fear over face masks, especially early in the pandemic was tied to the inconsistencies in policy and the lack of ubiquitous evidence. Should everyone wear a face mask and when should they wear it? Over the course of the pandemic, medical authorities sent confusing messages. Both the U.S. surgeon general and the Centers for Disease Control and Prevention exhorted Americans not to wear masks in January and February, then reversed themselves in April.

The purpose of the various mandates at first was mostly to protect others by ensuring the covering of the face of anyone who was infected. A study published in *Nature Medicine* in April looked at 246 people with acute upper respiratory illness and found that wearing a surgical mask did decrease spread of genetic material from respiratory viruses, including coronaviruses. The researchers concluded: "We also demonstrated the efficacy of surgical masks to reduce coronavirus detection and viral copies in large respiratory droplets and in aerosols. . . . This has important implications for control of COVID-19, suggesting that surgical face masks could be used by ill people to reduce onward transmission."

Yet another April study, published in the *Annals of Internal Medicine*, revealed that the force of sick patients' coughs could propel droplets through both surgical masks as well as cloth masks, so the mask as a barrier wasn't perfect.

What about asymptomatic patients? Transmission was certainly commonplace with COVID, but there was no exact science. The CDC based its revised mask recommendation on studies that found asymptomatic spread was far more common than had been thought, perhaps as much as 40 percent of cases. But there had been no exact studies on masks' effectiveness in preventing it. Although the coronavirus was highly contagious, it was still much less so than, say, measles, which could linger in the air for at least two hours after a cough or a sneeze. By contrast, the COVID-19 virus had not been proven to be aerosolized though there was certainly growing evidence that it could remain in the air too, though not nearly as long as measles. Coronaviruses also often entered the body through the eyes, and frequent hand and face washing, along with social distancing were just as important if not more than mask wearing.

Wearing a mask could provide a false sense of security, leading people to take fewer precautions. According to the World Health Organization, self-contamination and reuse and improper disposal of masks could also hinder their effectiveness and turn them into vehicles of spread.

Masks became a prop against our COVID fears, and the more worried we became, the more our society was shut down and damaged from COVID, the more one group lauded masks as the solution while the other stood in complete denial. No matter whether the masks were dirty or coughed in or hanging off your nose or chin, no matter whether a person leered up into your face or wiped the mask with dirty fingers, no matter what, the mask offered invulnerability. Whereas mask opponents derived their invulnerability from denial, as if flaunting their disregard of all precautions (many also didn't use hand sanitizer or physically distant) somehow protected them from infection. Surges of infection occurred as a result in Texas, Arizona, California, and Florida, for example, where bars, restaurants and beaches were open, and hospitals soon filled as the result of young people cavorting. Months of restraint led quickly to months of indiscretion, and the number of new cases in the U.S. surged in July and August to more than 50,000 per day, with hospitalizations increasing as a result. The cases tended to be milder because younger people didn't tend to get as sick as older people, especially those with other medical problems, but they still were subject to longer term sequelae, and the burden on the health care system grew.

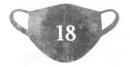

OPERATION
WARP SPEED

Being admitted to the White House these days included being nasally swabbed for COVID-19 and being issued a mask, if you didn't already have one. For this new reality to change, I suspected a widely used effective vaccine against the SARS COV 2 virus will have to become available. In the meantime, I was socially distanced from the president of the United States for an interview in the pillared walkway beside the Rose Garden.

He spoke about vaccines, and said that the "vaccines are doing well," but are "longer term." His immediate focus, he said, was on therapeutics including the anti-viral remdesivir, steroids, and antibodies against the virus. "If I had my choice of vaccines or therapeutics, give me therapeutics every time because I'd love to walk into a hospital and give everybody something and they start walking out in two days."

Unfortunately, though the current therapeutics were helpful, the clinical response was nowhere near this dramatic. The scientific community was right to continue to chase the holy grail of vaccines. The news the day of my interview was that the Pfizer/BioNTech vaccine had been contracted by Health and Human Services to provide 100 million doses for $2 billion. President Trump smiled and acknowledged this proudly. The vaccine utilizes messenger RNA, a genetic communicator, which works by informing our cells to make the same spike protein the virus has in order to cause an immune response against it. SARS COV 2, like many viruses, is composed of RNA, a single strand of unstable genetic material.

Vaccine research for COVID-19 was proceeding at a prodigious pace. Two messenger RNA vaccines, Pfizer/BioNTech and Moderna, had shown a robust immune response to the virus in early studies and were tolerated well, albeit with flu-like symptoms in a majority of cases. Both vaccines made substantial neutralizing antibodies which attack the spike protein on the virus, and both vaccines also made so-called "T" cells, immune warriors against viruses which augment the antibody response. Both vaccines had also protected non-human primates against the virus in challenge trials and both were now entering late stage trials.

A third high tech vaccine was even further along. The Oxford University/Astra Zeneca vaccine, which utilized a viral vector—a deactivated chimpanzee adenovirus—to deliver the genetic payload (resembles the spike protein of the virus) to trigger the immune response, may have completed clinical trials by late Fall.

And then there was the Johnson & Johnson adenovirus based vaccine, which was a few months behind the others, but had also shown promising results.

The dark horse in the race, with a powerful finishing kick perhaps, was an innovative vaccine produced by Novavax, where the spike protein was grown in insects, and when placed in human volunteers in early trials the amount of antibodies produced was an eight fold rise in neutralizing antibody titres. Novavax was also awarded $1.6 billion from the Trump Administration's Operation Warp Speed to produce 100 million doses.

Speaking of fear, in Russia a COVID-19 vaccine known as "Sputnik V" that had only been given to 76 people in early trials was approved for use in August, ahead of a planned late stage trial of 40,000 people. The vaccine utilized an adenovirus vector, like several other vaccines, and was created at the prestigious Gamaleya Institute, but hadn't been fully tested. Fear of the government itself might ensure enough compliance to overcome fear of an untested vaccine.

China too had several vaccines in late stage trials utilizing different genetic technologies, including one from CanSino Biologics.

This was the best of science both in terms of speed and skilled biotechnology. In the U.S., the Operation Warp Speed program was cutting corners only on the manufacturing side by the government buying hundreds of millions of doses in advance of any vaccine being approved. It was reassuring that vaccines had been in development previously for SARS and MERS, and that there were coronavirus vaccines in common use for animals.

But it would it would still be a monumental chore to convince a nervous public to take a new vaccine, even with mild side affects and even if the virus was still surging in the Winter. The involvement of the Department of Defense in a partnership with Health and Human Services was also likely to be reassuring when it came to distribution.

Still, these were all new technologies that had never been tried before which made them exciting, but unpredictable at the same time.

What remained to be seen is whether the vaccines would work and be well tolerated in the much larger numbers of volunteers (approximately 30,000) involved in Phase Three trials. Would there be enough virus around in the hot spots where the vaccines were being tested to conclude that they actually prevented you from becoming infected or decreased your symptoms if you did the way non-human primate studies had shown in several of the candidates? Could encountering the virus increase your side effects from the vaccine? Would more risky challenge trials, where the virus was deliberately given to those who have been vaccinated, have to be considered?

If and when a coronavirus vaccine was approved for use in humans, we would also need to overcome the compliance problem. Several polls suggested that a third to half of Americans would not take a COVID vaccine.

There was also significant COVID health care disparity and we needed to make sure the vaccine was freely available in socioeconomically disadvantaged communities where high risk groups for spreading and suffering severe cases of the virus predominated.

Dr. Jose Romero, head of the CDC's Advisory Committee on Immunization Practices suggested that minority groups get prioritized when it came to receiving a new vaccine against COVID-19. The committee agreed to prioritize essential workers, those with underlying conditions who put them at higher risk of complications, and those who lived in nursing homes and homeless shelters.

It was imperative that Black and Latino people be on this priority list. Not as a political statement to address our country's history of unequal care for minorities, though this continued to be an open wound, but because these groups had been infected with COVID-19 at three times the rate of white people, and have died nearly twice as frequently. In fact a recent study from Louisiana published in the New England Journal of Medicine revealed that 70 percent of those hospitalized for COVID-19 were Black. The lead author of this study, Dr. Eboni Price Haywood of Ochsner Health, told us in an interview on SiriusXM Doctor Radio that the reasons for this disparity were partly due to greater incidence of obesity, diabetes, hypertension, and kidney disease, later diagnosis because of inadequate access to care, jobs that put them at greater risk of acquiring COVID-19, and poorer living conditions. These were chronic problems but applied directly to COVID.

In medical school we learned to treat patients by problem and health risk, not by skin color. It meant showing respect and kindness to all patients. Distrust and mistreatment of course bred fear and non-compliance. The COVID pandemic racial disparities were deeply disturbing.

I was glad to see NIH director Dr. Francis Collins and CDC director Dr. Robert Redfield emphasizing the need for racial diversity in vaccine clinical trials at a Senate hearing. In order to gauge the effectiveness of vaccines we needed to test it equally on everyone, the essence of good science.

The pandemic started back in February in the U.S. accompanied by an ugly fear and targeting of Asian people. This target moved on to a fear of minorities as spreaders of the disease. We needed to accept the history of our unequal response and learn from it as a society. The pandemic needed to end by all of us coming together and protecting those most at risk by putting them at the front of the line to receive a vaccine. Equality was essential to public health. No time better to show our sense of fairness and propriety than in the middle of a massive pandemic.

It was also going to be necessary to overcome the fear of flu-like side effect once it became well known that a new vaccine caused them. The goal for me and other practicing physicians would be to convince people that fear of the virus should be greater than fear of the vaccine to prevent it. This would be easier to accomplish if clinical trials were fully completed before a vaccine became available and I was able to rely entirely on the science to promote vaccine compliance.

But was utilizing fear to overcome fear enough to overcome this much potential non-compliance? I had always relied on leaders to cement resolve and help me and other physicians to fight public worry. So in July, while I was interviewing President Trump, I brought him in on my concern and mentioned the non-compliance figure. Knowing about his history as a vaccine skeptic I took a chance and asked him, "as Commander-in-Chief and leader of the free world, would you consider being one of the first to take this vaccine to send a message to the American public?"

His willingness surprised me. This was the same president who had showed some reluctance to wear a mask even as the virus continued to spread and it became clear that a mask played at least some role in slowing it down.

"Well you know the way it works. If I'm the first one, they'll say he's so selfish he wanted to get the vaccine first. And then other people would say, hey, that's a very brave thing to do. I would absolutely if they wanted me to and if they thought it was right. I'd take it first or I'd take it last. . . . If I take it first, and if I take it . . . if I don't take it, they'll say he doesn't believe in the program. But whatever I think is best, whatever we all agree is best, I would certainly do that."

"I'll make you a deal," I said. "I'll take it and then you."

"We will take it together," Trump agreed.

"That's right," I said.

"Good," said the president.

His willingness was a big victory for vaccine compliance and overcoming fear. If a COVID vaccine emerged the president (if he was still president by then) had declared he will join me at the front of the line to take it. Millions of vaccine skeptics would see this and hopefully take it too.

THE POLITICS OF FEAR: MENTAL HEALTH AND SCHOOLS

Fear of the virus translated readily into a cycle of worry. We clung to fear props, false gods against this fear. Fear leaders, when effective, helped to reassure us and allay these fears, at least temporarily. But the problem was that they were too often inconsistent and ineffective, especially as the virus continued to spread around the country and the hot spots shifted from the Northeast to the South and West to the Midwest. Rising new case numbers of over 50,000 per day scared people throughout the summer of 2020, even though the death rate didn't rise correspondingly and stayed around 1,000 nationwide. Everyone focused on these case numbers and lost perspective on their meaning. For example, in a state like Florida, a hot spot, was consistently reporting more than a 10 percent test positivity rate through July, with 20 percent in some areas including Miami. That sounded incredibly scary, but consider what that actually meant. If you thought you could be positive or at risk and went for a test, there was a 90 percent chance you would be negative. In New York, where the case positivity rate hovered at around one percent through the summer, this meant that there was a 99 percent chance that if you were tested you would be negative. And yet, fear clouded perception and New Yorkers (as I can attest) continued to feel they were far more at risk than the statistics showed. This fear could be useful if it led to caution, but many were reckless about physical distancing and wore their masks (if at all) down around their chins as more of a statement than an actual public health measure.

Meanwhile, the news media drove ratings with mainly bad news, so that when the case positivity rate fell below 7 percent in California in mid August and below 8 percent in Florida, and the new case numbers fell dramatically in both states, the news barely reported it.

The fear and foreboding combined with continued behavioral restrictions to create a severe mental health crisis in our country, The entire country experienced an adjustment disorder as unemployment remained elevated and many people stayed in their cocoons. Businesses like restaurants and movie theaters and gyms were in deep trouble all across the country.

And yet, by late August the case numbers and hospitalization numbers and death numbers dropped precipitously. Public health measures certainly played a role, though full lockdowns were unbelievably primitive and barely worked when there was already a lot of virus in the area. They were especially faulty when they weren't accompanied by consistent travel restrictions and screenings to help protect regions like New York, where the case numbers had dropped precipitously and only 0.6 percent were testing positive by late August.

By late August, numbers in the big new hot spots were dropping, while the economic continued to flounder because of all the continuing restrictions. On August 25th, the new case numbers for the U.S. were once again below 35,000 and the number of deaths below 350. New case numbers and hospitalization numbers were dropping precipitously in Florida, Texas, and California. We were clearly heading in the right direction.

But why? Was it all compliance and public health? That was certainly a big part of it. But there was something else to consider amidst all the hype and hysteria. Perhaps the virus might be burning itself out, ravaging one region before moving on. If this were true, there could be several reasons for this. First, many people had developed antibodies to the virus who weren't aware of it, especially in low socioeconomic regions where the virus was most common. Second, a huge piece of immunity was T cell (immune warrior cells) and T cell memory, which wasn't being reported. Third, there was likely some cross immunity from other coronaviruses, and fourth, there were pockets of people who might not be susceptible to SARS COV 2 at all.

When this was all over, public health officials and local politicians in certain states were sure to take a victory lap, but it might well not be fully warranted.

Dr. Scott Atlas of the Hoover Institute at Stanford University told me he believed that the virus was slowing down because a much higher percentage of people had immunity to it (mostly T cells) than we realized. I felt that the virus might have saturated certain regions in terms of who was most susceptible or who had partial protection from prior exposure to other coronaviruses. Either way, in late August it appeared that we might finally be getting some control over the virus, as the overall new daily case numbers in the U.S. were consistently below 50,000, most days under 40,000 and perhaps more importantly, the hospitalization numbers were declining as well.

Arizona seemed to be making a good case for the positive impact of public health measures on viral spread. One of the first states to emerge from lockdown in May, they had experienced a burgeoning of cases in June, only to reclose bars, gyms, restaurants, movie theaters, restrict large gatherings, what I liked to call a laser or surgical lockdown, with emphasis on the places (mostly indoors) where spread was the most likely. There was no official mask mandate, but most counties had them.

Now in August they had seen a drop-off of cases and there was a controversy about re-opening again, but Governor Arizona Doug Ducey held firm this time, and moved more slowly regarding reopening. This was clearly a wise decision.

People everywhere worried about the Fall, with flu season coming and the possibility that there could be an even further increase of COVID cases. I started giving out flu shots in late August this year, and I was heartened by the very mild flu season in Australia, which was six months ahead of us and tended to predict what we would be facing. There was also the possibility that all the social distancing, masking, hand washing, and disinfecting was being put to good use against the flu, a seemingly much less contagious virus thanSARS COV 2. Still, in the absence of a significant mutation, "second wave" for COVID appeared to be yet another fear mongering term promoted for political reasons, including undermining the Trump administration's efforts. Second wave appeared to be a fiction at this point, despite the fact that respiratory viruses were more easily transmissible indoors and at times of low humidity.

SCHOOLS

Functioning schools are part of the backbone of our society. But as we approached the Fall of 2020, schools were still mostly on line, which deeply damaged socialization especially in younger children and led to a further fracturing of our culture. Especially for lower socio-economic groups, schools were at the center of mental health care, nutrition, vaccination compliance, and even making sure that child abuse was reported. The shuttering of schools across the country had a deep impact on the psyche of not just students, but also teachers and parents. Solo on line learning disrupted everyone's lives.

Teachers across the country resisted the call to return, afraid for their own health, concerned that none of the proposed plans to ensure physical distancing, masking, and rapid testing had actually been instituted. Where were the nurses needed to screen everyone for symptoms? Temperature taking wasn't enough—frequently COVID presented with nuanced various symptoms including slight cough, sore throat, shortness of breath, chest pain, diarrhea, muscle aches, loss of sense of taste or smell, or simply fatigue. Teachers were concerned that they could get sick, spread it among themselves, end up hospitalized. Their concern was legitimate, especially when plans to protect them were not in place.

Several physicians told me their teacher/patients were already asking for doctors notes in August.

In New York, the United Federation of Teachers Solidarity caucus opposed Governor Cuomo and Mayor Di Blasio's plan to reopen New York City Schools two to three days a week and asked for the immediate resignation of School Chancellor Richard Carranza.

The forces of fear were fighting (and winning in most places) against the decreasing amount of virus and the needs of the children. The New York Times published a frightening map suggesting that a vast majority of counties across the country would open schools with a high risk of a child testing positive. I felt this was hyperbole, but it would be accepted as fact among the left leaning intelligentsia.

But it wasn't all hypothetical. Across the country, from Nebraska to Tennessee to Georgia to Alabama, school closures followed students and staff becoming infected. These responses were based more on fear than on science. Better to reform practices if possible than to quickly close schools.

Meanwhile, multiple studies conducted in South Korea, Europe and Australia that showed that younger children were much less likely to spread the virus to adults, and had a very low percentage of severe illness and death themselves. In fact, according to CDC, less than 600 children under the age of 18 had been hospitalized since the beginning of the pandemic to the end of July.

In late August, CDC director Dr. Robert Redfield cited a new CDC report looking at 666 childcare centers in Rhode Island which reported very limited transmission of COVID-19 among children and staff. Redfield said that as schools reopen, if more than 90 percent of Americans adhere to mask wearing, social distancing, and hand hygiene, he believed the outbreak could be brought under control.

I was among those who pushed for elementary schools to open especially in non hot spots. I was completely aware that fear of the virus as well as fear of lawsuits would lead to school closure if even one student got sick, but I felt we had to try. The collateral damage of school closure was far greater than the risk of the virus itself. In fact, the CDC studied mental health problems the last week of June, and found that 40 percent of U.S. adults (especially younger adults) suffering from mental health problems and substance abuse associated with COVID-19. For children, the problem was even worse. School closures were part of the reason, placing a heavy wait on our society.

In terms of testing, I believed that surveillance testing was best—test all incoming students and staff initially for COVID, but then use targeted testing to figure out the percentage of positivity and react accordingly. This approach would decrease the fear and hysteria of schools reopening. The goal was to protect high risk groups among both teachers and students, while encouraging the school to continue function.

I was proud of the school all my children had attended, Horace Mann School, a top private school in the Bronx, because it devised an elaborate system that I thought would work. First, they began with tents outside for the initial weeks in September, where physical distancing was easier and where the virus (if present), would be much less likely to spread. They had nurses to screen students and faculty, testing capabilities, and a plan to isolate possible cases. It made sense to me to test everyone coming in, followed by surveillance testing to determine the rate of positivity, while of course testing all who were symptomatic automatically. All the procedures that teachers across the country were demanding were in place at Horace Mann. The school would start, across all divisions, with a five day week.

Of course there was no guarantee that any of this would work if the coronavirus returned in great numbers to the New York City area, a possibility all the hospitals including mine were preparing for. My son Sam, entering his sophomore year in high school at Horace Mann, said to me wisely, "at least we are getting to meet our teachers and they are getting to meet us. So even if we end up on line, we will know them and they will know us."

UNIVERSITIES HAD AN advantage. They had built-in quarantine situations and could isolate patients and even quarantine the entire university if necessary. Cornell University decided to bring its students back to campus, and most of the student body planned to be there until they cancelled their quarantine options in mid August, which had students scrambling for accommodations. Duke brought its student body back for in person classes too, as did Notre Dame, starting off with a positive paradigm, testing close to 12,000 people before allowing students on campus, and just 33 tested positive, less than 0.5 percent. Unfortunately, from August 6th to August 14th, 29 cases were positive (8 percent of the 348 tests conducted, close to half on the football program and most of the rest on symptomatic students or their contacts). The university reported that many of the cases were traced to an off-campus party where students were not compliant with masks or physical distancing. The university vowed to try to stay open and increase its focus on compliance. But by August 17th they were reporting a whopping 19% positivity rate and 147 cases total. Notre Dame felt compelled to go fully on-line, at least for two weeks. I wasn't optimistic that they would return to in-person classes any time soon.

Meanwhile, Ohio State opened too, also with an extensive testing program in place, and fared better at the outset, whereas University of North Carolina at Chapel Hill echoed the Notre Dame experience, with four clusters of cases in the early going. And on August 17th they too capitulated to the pressure and went fully on-line only. Their quarantine center was full.

CDC had strict guidelines in place, but these were difficult for colleges to enforce, and it began to seem inevitable that most if not all of our universities would end up on-line if case clusters continued to occur.

Harvard went to an on line model early, despite the fact that Massachusetts had few cases. Brown (my alma mater) and Columbia and many other colleges across the country soon followed suit, motivated by fear and legal and medical ramifications if the virus continued to spread. I was deeply disappointed that my alma mater, Brown, joined many other colleges and went to on line learning alone. Especially since the numbers were very low in Rhode Island. Many students took gap years rather than pay full tuition for online classes and planned to travel around the country, potentially spreading virus from one hot spot to another.

The discussion about schools often centered around a potential vaccine. Some schools said would only reopen once a vaccine became available.

But would this be the magic bullet that schools needed? Would the fear of the virus by overcome by a vaccine, or would the speed of Operation Warp Speed, leading to an FDA approved and rapidly manufactured vaccine cause its own fears which led to non-compliance? For this easily transmissible a virus, it was clear that a majority of the population would have to take an effective vaccine to slow the virus down, creating enough "herd immunity" to overcome fears of the virus at schools.

In the meantime, what did we have to slow our fears? Washing our hands, disinfecting surfaces, keeping a physical distance, and the icing on the physical-distance cake, wearing a mask and wearing it properly. Many experts were doubtful that young children would be compliant with masks at schools, and besides, masks were not the whole public health cake, too many felt a false sense of security wearing them.

We all held our breath and waited for a vaccine, and while I advocated for the reopening of schools, I knew I would be defeated in most places, not by the virus itself, but by fear of lawsuits or the occurrence of even a single mild case.

The mental health of our children was at stake, but we were not nearly as afraid of their damaged psyches as we should have been.

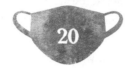

MORE FEAR
PROPS

Over the summer, China was testing frozen food for the coronavirus, and discovered it on Ecuadorian shrimp and chicken wings from Brazil. This might have been considered ultimate justice, were the exporters of the virus to the world to be receiving it back on food imports, except that from a public health point of view it was an extremely unlikely source of contagion. Even the World Health Organization said so, though of course difficult to believe anything they said at this point.

Still, the science backed this up. The vast majority of transmission was via respiratory droplets, with the fecal/oral route a possible secondary route. A study from Nebraska Med did show that the coronavirus was found on multiple surfaces in the rooms where the quarantined patients from the Diamond Princess ship had stayed, though no one had gotten sick from these surfaces, including me and my team from Tucker Carlson Tonight, who had travelled to the Quarantine Center in late February and spent time in the same room with the health care workers there.

Which is not to say that disinfection wasn't an essential part of trying to contain the pandemic.

Meanwhile, over in New Zealand, a country that had effectively prevented the virus from entering by locking down in advance and cutting off travel, suddenly reported 30 cases in August which appeared to center around an Americold food storage facility. It was far more likely that workers on a freight ship or at the port had spread the infections rather than food being the source, still, panic spread and the entire country locked down. In Auckland, a city of 1.7 million people, you were unable to leave your home again except for an essential reason. I had been a fan of the initial lockdown in New Zealand, because it was coupled by isolating the island, but the move in response to the very small outbreak was clearly hysteria-driven.

I told people it was perfectly okay to eat ice cream from the freezer without boiling it, and to have chicken wings, though it was of course better to cook them first, it was more to kill E Coli than any coronavirus.

FEAR PROPS—TESTING

Speaking of fiascos, back in February, when COVID-19 first appeared in the U.S., a small outbreak in the state of Washington, the Centers for Disease Control and Prevention sent around 100 test kits, most of which turned out to be faulty. The test itself was the gold standard Polymerase Chain Reaction, the gold standard, and Dr. Robert Redfield, director of CDC was correct to point out to me in an interview on Doctor Radio that this had been developed for SARS COV 2 rapidly, but this paled in comparison to the production problems. In fact, we were never even close to keeping up with the spread of this virus, were never able to contact trace properly or isolate and quarantine the necessary people to prevent spread. This incompetence spread fear along with virus as people got sick and flooded hospitals, first here in the Northeast and later in the South and West. Even after Admiral Giroir, Deputy Health and Human Services Secretary for Health took over the program in mid March, the delays continued. It was months before nasal swabs (which required less personal protective equipment) were tested and used instead of the more cumbersome uncomfortable nasopharyngeal swabs, and it wasn't until August before rapid test results began to be more uniformly available and saliva testing (which might be self administered) became available. All of this delay spread virus and fear. Over 70 million tests had been conducted by August, but many of these tests were too delayed to be useful in preventing spread.

By August, rapid antigen testing began to become commonly available, months after both Dr. Giroir and Dr. Fauci of NIH told me they would be. Antigen testing, though not quite as accurate as the PCR test, was very useful, as with flu, in testing a large group of people (pool testing), or in surveiling a large group to determine the rate of positivity, swooping in with more tests if that rate went up. It was unfortunate that by the time this test became commonplace, we already had over 5 million documented cases in the U.S., and as the CDC indicated, the true number was probably far greater.

We also hadn't reached the point by August where we had standardized antibody testing and we still didn't know if a positive test indicated true immunity or for that matter how long this immunity lasted.

All of this uncertainty spread fear, and distrust of our public health leadership. I was not used to the idea of a public health disaster of this magnitude where the CDC was not riding shot gun, calling the shots, advising the states. Dr. Fauci and Dr. Birx (coronavirus task force co-ordinator) and Dr. Giroir had assumed this role, but historically it should have been CDC director Redfield's position. Center for Disease Control and Prevention—the name says it all.

By late August, when testing was widespread and over 75 million tests had been done since March, there was still a several day delay in obtaining results in many places. The faster the results came back, the less frightened we were. We were able to use a negative test to reassure ourselves and a positive result to cause us to isolate ourselves and not subject others to a contagious powerful virus. Of course simply knowing these results didn't automatically mean a person was going to behave appropriately.

Also by August, saliva tests were being approved by the FDA that held the promise of home testing. This would definitely provide an additional means of reassurance. I was in favor of widespread testing, and the rapid antigen (viral protein) tests like we had with the flu were finally becoming available. They weren't always as accurate as the PCR test which could be a problem, but they were cheaper and could be used in bulk, a process known as pool testing, where entire populations at risk were tested at once and those who are positive were then separated from the group. This provided a practical way for a school or a business to remain open and calm.

When I interviewed President Trump in late July he pointed out that excess testing created an avenue for fear and worry even if it was essential for good public health. "And to me, if every time you test, you find a case and, you know, it gets reported in the news. We found more cases. If instead of 50 (million), we did 25 would have half the number of cases. . . . You know, we have so many more tests than any other country by far. . . . We're spending a lot of money on massive testing and I'm okay with it."

In fact, the pandemic was surging in other parts of the world in July and August, especially Latin America. Brazil had the second largest number of cases after the U.S. with over 3 million, and a fraction of the testing was being done, so the real numbers were actually much higher. The death rate was also much higher than the U.S., with 250,000 deaths throughout Latin America and the Caribbean. India was another burgeoning hot spot, also with over 3 million cases, though the death rate seemed lower, with about 60,000 cases total. India, though testing more than Brazil, was still testing far less than the U.S. Political battles, vulnerable communities, poor health care, and dense populations were all reasons for the rapid spread and poor outcomes.

Here in the U.S., there was a developing controversy regarding how much testing should be done and who should get it. In late August the CDC released new guidelines NOT to test people who were asymptomatic but had been in brief close contact with those who were sick with COVID.

Many public health officials across the country challenged this, saying it made no sense, and questioned the political motives. Surely testing of all contacts made sense, especially since asymptomatic spread was so common. I spoke about this to CDC director Dr. Robert Redfield, and he tried to clarify CDC's position. he said the purpose of the guidance was to make sure that testing was tied to the ability by public health officials to actually trace contacts. i gave as an example my asymptomatic patient who had spent hours exposed to his superintendent (who then tested positive for COVID) three days before—he had been working in my patient's apartment—and Redfield agreed he should be immediately tested.

At the same time, FDA issued an Emergency Use Authorization for Abbott's $5, fifteen minute, point of care antigen (protein test) for the SARS COV 2 virus, which clinical studies had shown to be at least 97 percent accurate. When the patient had symptoms and had a high viral load in their nostrils. The platform was called BinaxNow, it used lateral flow technology that didn't rely on elaborate lab equipment or CLIA safety approvals, and it had potential for home use and Iphone linkup where the results of the test would be beamed to you almost instantly.

Redfield agreed with me that this was a huge potential game changer, He said it would change the focus to screening large numbers of patients. Abbott planned to ship many millions of tests in September, and 50 million in October. HHS contracted for 150 million tests overall. This exciting advance, if coupled with another test (still to be developed), to accurately screen asymptomatic patients at risk, meant that everyone at risk could be tested regularly.

In the meantime, it was clear to me that regardless of your interpretation of guidelines, everyone who had potentially come in contact with a COVID patient should be tested, as contact tracing was a proven public health concept, and of course everyone who was positive or became symptomatic should immediately be isolated from the group and quarantined, decreasing the potential for spread. Schools or places of business should not automatically be closed because of a positive case, and fear needed to be treated and controlled.

FEAR PROPS—IMMUNITY

One of the greatest causes of uncertainty over the COVID-19 pandemic was the recurrent notion that perhaps there was no lasting immunity and you could get reinfected. I must say that I never believed it, which doesn't mean that the public didn't worry and that the notion didn't unsettle people further. The reason I was slow to subscribe to this theory was because 1—SARS COV 2 was a lot more like the first SARS virus than the common cold, where a lasting immunity didn't occur. 2—according to a top infectious diseases expert told me that when patients with COVID were recovering in the hospital they showed immunity afterwards even if they had conditions (hypogammaglobulinemia) where they didn't make antibodies. 3—top vaccine candidates including the Pfizer/BioNtech, Moderna, Oxford/Astra Zeneca, Nanovax, and Johnson & Johnson all showed a robust neutralizing (against the spike protein on the virus) antibody response.

The missing link was T cells, the body's immune warriors against viruses, and studies (including a landmark study published in August in the journal CELL), showed a robust T Cell response.

Also in August, an unusual study from the Greninger Lab at the University of Washington published in *Nature* provided the first direct evidence that the antibodies against the new coronavirus protected people from reinfection. A crew of a fishing vessel were tested for antibodies and 120 out of 122 were found to be negative for SARS COV 2. But an outbreak hit the ship and 104 crew members were infected. All three of the crew who had antibodies were spared.

Earlier in the pandemic, this news might have gone a long way towards calming public fears. Not only was it clear evidence that once you got COVID and got over it you were immune to getting it again, at least for a period of time, but it also provided indirect evidence that vaccines that show a strong antibody response against the virus would work.

Unfortunately, as I will address in the next chapter, by the time this news came out it was buried under the constant onslaught of news about the presidential election, only a few months away. The Democrats were focused on the supposed failings of the Trump administration's handling of the COVID pandemic, despite all the movement on supplies, treatments, and vaccines with a highly evolved public/private partnership. Former Vice President Biden and others called out President Trump for a lack of strong leadership, leaving too much to the states including policies on masking, and for a delayed response in testing.

Even if they were right, the result of all this flame throwing was to create more divisiveness and more fear.

FEAR LEADERS
IN THE TIME OF COVID

The frightened public looks for fear guides especially during times of perceived danger. During my lifetime the national fear quotient has never been higher than during the coronavirus pandemic, except perhaps during the height of the Cold War in the 1960s. Then the strident sonorous proclamations soothed America and carried us through the fear and foreboding. As a young child I was too young to be thinking the world could end at any given nuclear moment, or perhaps that was a great lesson for me to learn, not a descendant of a Holocaust family but one whose great grandparents had had their heads smashed in by the Cossacks in a bloody Bialystok pogrom in 1903.

In 2001, we gained another fear guide where we were least expecting one. President George W. Bush's pausing and fumbling when hearing of the 9/11 attacks while reading My Pet Goat to a group of first graders transformed overnight to his fiery megaphoned proclamation on top of the car at Ground Zero;

"I want you all to know that America today is on bended knee in prayer for the people whose lives were lost here, for the workers who work here, for the families who mourn. This nation stands with the good people of New York City and New Jersey and Connecticut as we mourn the loss of thousands of our citizens. I can hear you! I can hear you! The rest of the world hears you. And the people who knocked these buildings down will hear all of us soon."

This moment soon transformed itself into the global war on terror, leading to two wars and great loss of national treasure, as I have discussed in this book. But for at least three years following 9/11, it galvanized America behind its leader, as we siphoned his personal courage to help us overcome our fear of terrorism.

Later, I met President Bush, after he was out of office, in 2012 at Palo Duro Canyon State Park just outside of Amarillo, Texas, for a 100 kilometer mountain bike ride on the toughest mountain bike trails in the country.

Why was I there?

I was covering the event (second annual) for Fox News.

How did this come to happen?

I had asked Dana Perino, Bush's former press secretary, who I worked with at Fox, for an introduction to—not the former president—but to the White House doctor who had taken care of him, Dr. Tubbs.

But Dana asked Bush himself if I could interview him about his health and he told her to ask me if I rode a mountain bike.

"Tell him I rode my bicycle across the U.S. twice when I was a kid.

Evidently, this impressed the former president, because he invited me on this mountain bike ride and said if I could finish it he would grant me an exclusive interview, something he rarely did. I was inspired and hauled my road bike out, having barely ridden it since the crowning achievement of my youth.

20 miles a day for over a month later, I was ready, though I still didn't know how to ride a mountain bike. On the trail, Bush assigned one of his mountain bike coaches, who as it happens had won an Olympic gold medal in off road biking, to teach me the art in two hours, including how to get in and out of clipless pedals. She warned me about cactus and rattlesnakes out on the trail.

It was 105 degrees. Luckily, I had purchased one of those camelbacks that held a gallon of water and I drank almost every drop of it. I fell twenty seven times, rode over a rattlesnake, but managed to finish the first days 17 mile assignment. I was sore, and I would be picking cactus out of my butt for the next month, but I finished in the lower third of the pack, but not near the bottom. The last mile of the trail there was an ambulance circling overhead like a vulture, and seven people were taken to the hospital, three with heart attacks.

The veterans themselves, over twenty in total (the entire group including support staff and active duty officers, Navy Seals, Green Berets, and a medical team), all finished. They rode in formation, helping each other up when they fell. Some amputees rode special bicycles outfitted for prostheses, while for others the wounds were invisible. All benefitted from the camaraderie, the shared purpose, and the bonding experience with their former commander in chief.

Word reached him about my experience and he decided to grant me an interview right then. We stood together outside a lodge where the ride concluded. He wasn't anything like what I expected him to be like from media coverage. He exuded warmth, ease with himself, and a canny intelligence.

"I had very low expectations, but you exceeded them," the former president said. And in a moment that inspired me for years afterward he told me that what mattered to him the most was personal toughness, never giving up, and I had shown that quality. I was invited on the W100K every year going forward (future rides took place on his ranch in Crawford, Texas.

As inspired as I was, I knew this wasn't about me, it was about the Vets, and about the former president's personal leadership quality, his own personal form of toughness that had brought our country through the early part of the 21st century. Whether or not you approved of the Iraq War or not, it was clear to me, when I met him, that Bush was a deeply feeling man who inspired those around him to accept him as their leader.

"We can't possibly relate to see what its like to see a friend killed in combat," he said to me on the W100K a few years later. "But there are others who can."

PRESIDENT TRUMP HAS definite leadership qualities and a personal charm and charisma which he manifested to me in person, but unfortunately he did not always express a unified message that would have inspired the bipartisan masses to automatically follow him during the terrible days of the COVID pandemic. He did play an effective role as Anti-Fear Monger-in Chief throughout the Spring, though many took this as under-reacting to the risk. Certainly, he couldn't be blamed for all the mixed messaging and the delay in identifying or isolating cases. The CDC deeply underestimated COVID-19, and even if Trump wasn't the cause, he was held responsible.

Dr. Anthony Fauci, head of the National Institute of Allergy and Infectious Diseases, soon took the lead, but though he took this virus very seriously, his messaging also wasn't consistent, and as a virologist rather than a strict public health or health policy expert, he didn't always calculate the cost of strict strategies such as multiple statewide lockdowns.

Trump's brazen unfettered qualities emanated from a personal courage which was evident to me when I first met him. He was at ease with himself. He took the virus seriously, held daily press briefings throughout the Spring, and was very keen on the public-private partnership that finally accelerated testing, led to a prodigious effort for treatments and an unprecedented push for a vaccine (Operation Warp Speed). Trump's business skills were certainly extremely useful in accelerating the crucial biotechnology. By mid August, the president had invoked the Defense Production Act 78 times to provide masks, personal protective equipment, vaccine and accelerated testing development. There was no shortage of ventilators or PPE over the summer as the pandemic continued. And many other businesses didn't have to be asked, they just stepped up to the plate into a climate that encouraged co-operation.

Unfortunately, the CDC was still slow to react, and CDC Director Dr. Robert Redfield and Dr. Anthony Fauci director of the National Institute of Allergies and Infectious Diseases told me in interviews on Doctor Radio SiriusXM that they had relied on good relationships with top Chinese scientists at the beginning and that this information had helped guide them. Unfortunately, this information turned out to be faulty and suppressed and it was only after the fact when we began seeing patients here that we quickly found out how easily transmissible the virus was, and how it caused a multi-system inflammation beyond just the lungs, causing blood clotting and affecting the endothelial lining of blood vessels.

This lack of knowledge, and rapid spread without the CDC tests necessary to diagnose and isolate cases, or to do adequate contact tracing, had spread both fear and virus at the onset of the pandemic. The horses were long out of the barn and the Trump administration had to play catchup.

And after it became clear that the coronavirus had already spread throughout communities in the United States, Dr. Fauci in particular began to support extensive lockdowns and make dire predictions, both of which strangled our economy, spread more fear and foreboding, and undermined the president's more upbeat approach. They clearly had some value in terms of slowing the spread of the virus, but at tremendous cost.The perceived division between Fauci and the president, and later Dr. Birx and the president grew, when on August 2nd she said on CNN, "what we are seeing today is different from March and April. It is extraordinarily widespread. It's into the rural as well as urban areas." This provoked the president into a retaliatory tweet. "In order to counter Nancy (Pelosi), Deborah took the bait and hit us. Pathetic."

Unfortunately, the friction and division between Trump and his advisors spread more fear. I tended to blame the advisors more for it because I felt it was their job to differ with the president in private meetings, not on television.

THIS DIVISION CREATED an opening for opponents to step up as fear leaders. Here in New York, it began with Governor Cuomo who was strong at each press conference and speech, lobbying publically for 30,000 ventilators (most of which turned out to be unnecessary, and then taking credit for leading New York out of the woods when the case numbers and deaths from COVID dropped. While it was true that New York's hospitals rose to the challenge and the governor was a charismatic leader during this time, the presence of the USNS Comfort (sent by President Trump) also provided comfort worthy of its name even though it saw very few patients, and the Javits Center temporary field hospital which did see 1100 patients from late March until early May also reassured people that there was a functioning safety net here in New York.

It was clear that compliance with social distancing, masking, and across the board lockdown of most businesses, restaurants, bars, schools, gyms, hair salons, etc. was a major reason for the improvement even though it badly damaged the economy and psyche of the city. By July and August, less than 1 percent of those tested for COVID-19 were positive.

On the other hand, Cuomo received a lot of criticism for allowing a statute to remain on the books until May which compelled nursing homes to readmit patients who were COVID-19 positive, without the ability to properly isolate them, leading to over 7,000 deaths. It also turned out that he greatly exaggerated the number of ventilators we needed, the real number was closer to 6,000 (as a top level HHS official informed me), and Cuomo ended up giving unused ventilators away to other states. In the end, he wasn't the fear leader he appeared to be at first, even though New York was in much better shape COVID-wise in the summer than it had been in the Spring. Batting away the virus was also accompanied by a mass exodus from Manhattan.

FORMER VICE PRESIDENT Joe Biden ran for president on a big government platform that indicated that he wanted to play a much larger national role in controlling the pandemic, including a national mask mandate for everyone who was "outside." I felt this restriction could spread more panic, even if it were very useful inside businesses or restaurants, imagine if it were applied to those who were nowhere near anyone else. As I discussed in another chapter, masks were a big part of the politics of COVID fear. Although they were clearly very useful, and population studies on COVID showed effectiveness at decreasing spread, mask science was still evolving. And exactly how protective was a mask if a person was leering up into your face with one or wearing in over their chin or not cleaning it properly? Too many masks wearers had a false sense of security that they were fully protected against COVID.

Plus, there was a politics of fear that was steeped in the hypocrisy of a party that obsessed on mask wearing on the one hand but on the other promoted protests and riots that could easily spread the virus if there was any in the crowd. This was a contradiction in any fear leader who was on the one hand claiming that public health was all that mattered but on the other allowing a first amendment exception (churches and free speech not included) that put that at risk. Inconsistencies bred fear.

I was also concerned about the politics of fear as it applied to the health care system in general. Biden had talked about bringing back the individual mandate of Obamacare and creating a public option to buy in to Medicare. This was designed of course to reassure people that they had coverage while at the same time creating further revenue for the insurance companies and more government control. But if there was one thing the pandemic had exposed it was our problems on the supply side, with inadequate personal protective equipment or hazard pay for hospitals, doctors, nurses, or emergency personnel. There was also the need for private insurance (other than Obamacare) to pay for the amazing research that was going on for treatments and vaccines. Health and Human Services meanwhile provided reimbursement to health care providers and facilities for testing and treatment of COVID for the uninsured, so COVID claims were covered.

So Biden's talk of mandating expanded health coverage was occurring at the wrong time, preying on public fears without in any way helping with the pandemic itself. At the same time, especially by late August, it was hardly a given that superimposed federal mandates were the answer. By August 20th, the overall case numbers were again below 25,000, the new case rate was dropping in Florida and California, with the case positivity rate being down to 6.6% in California and 8 percent in Florida. New York remained very low, with only 600 new cases that day, and only 19 in Maine. It was deeply unsettling to consider what a nationwide lockdown under Biden could do at this point to states with few cases. Children not getting dental or eye care, not receiving their vaccinations or proper nutrition. School re-opening was a major priority, but seemed less likely under a restrictive Biden approach. He planned daily briefings on COVID, expanded testing, and a more unified national policy, which could have an upside but also a serious downside if it was applied across the board.

On the other hand, during his acceptance speech for the Democratic Nomination, Biden projected strength and leadership, which was exactly what we needed. He talked about compassion and bringing us back from the darkness. This was what we needed to hear.

On a personal level, Biden had suffered greatly in his life, having lost his first wife Neilia and his 13 month old daughter Naomi in a fatal car crash in 1972. His two sons, Beau and Hunter, were injured in the crash too. Joe Biden said he briefly considered suicide. He had just been elected senator and in fact he took his oath of office from Beau's hospital room. Many years later, in 2015, Biden suffered through his son Beau's death from brain cancer.

During the Democratic National Convention, watching Biden speak, I could see the toughness and the courage that came from soldiering on after horrific tragedies. This courage built personal strength, and could also be a fulcrum for people trying to gather strength from leaders during a time of great crisis. With this speech Biden was setting himself up as a fear leader for COVID.

WE NEEDED FEAR guides, because in the midst of a massive pandemic, fear and hysteria over that pandemic were occurring at the same time. Public health measure were being compromised by both hysteria and denial. When we are afraid, fear hijacks our brain and we don't think rationally. Fear guides can help us through this.

One such guide was the U.S. Surgeon General, Dr. Jerome Michael Adams, who told me on Doctor Radio on SiriusXM that one of the lessons we'd learned from COVID was that "the world is a lot smaller than what we'd realized. What happens in China effects what is going to happen in Billings Montana. What happens in New York City is eventually going to affect what happens in my home town of Fishers, Indiana. And so we need to understand infectious diseases whether its COVID or whether its Ebola or whether its Zika don't respect state lines and don't respect incomes and in many cases don't discriminate based on any measure. All of us are at risk and are no more than a car trip or a plane ride away from these diseases."

Adams said that health starts in communities, that only 20 percent of our health is determined by access to traditional health care, a doctor, nurse, hospital, or clinic. 80 percent of our health, he said, is determined by transportation, safe and affordable housing, a job that pays a living wage and doesn't put you in harms way, and by access to child care. "COVID has brought all of these social determinants and pre existing social conditions to light in terms of who is most at risk for getting this disease. . . . We really are all in this together. What one person does whether its wearing a mask, or smoking a cigarette in public, or speeding down the highway, it impacts all of us. Either in the near term or in the long term. So we all really need to band together. One of the most challenging things is—this is a one in a century public health crisis. By any measure. But there's no page in the pandemic playbook for an impeachment trial, for a presidential election, for a social justice movement the likes of which we haven't seen in half a century. . . . So we always need to come back to the fact that we are all in this together and if we put health and public health first then that will help all the other things play out in a way that is most beneficial. But if we put these other things ahead of coming together for public health, then we are all going to lose."

Adams was a natural leader against fear. By his words and hearing the quiet passion in his voice, I could tell how much he cared. He said that we had to answer people's questions, to not make "health conversations into political conversations or us versus them conversations." Adams said, "people need to know that you care before they care what you know."

After the interview I knew that we had the right Surgeon General in place for this pandemic, to help us all fight our fears.. I only wished he could have a larger role or be more visible.

A MAJOR PROBLEM with pandemic messaging was that our politicians/leaders were not scientists or physicians, and our public health experts and virologists were not leaders. I had known Anthony Fauci, Director of the National Institute of Allergy and Infectious Diseases for many years, and at the beginning of the coronavirus outbreak I interviewed him for Doctor Radio and for Fox News and suggested him for several programs. He soon warned about this virus, and about the old-fashioned public health measures that were needed to try to contain it. He was a top virologist who always seemed to have the interest of the public at heart, and was especially convincing when it came to vaccines, somewhat less so when he spoke of lockdowns without always mentioning the limitations when the virus was already spreading throughout a community as well as the enormous collateral damage (including anxiety).

Scott Atlas MD was a different kind of fear leader, in that he came from the emotionless world of data crunching. He was added to the coronavirus task force in August, as a special advisor to the president, and he quickly took center stage alongside the president, calming public fears. While he lacked Dr. Birx's (coronavirus task force co-ordinator) or Dr. Fauci's (head of the National Institute of Allergy and Infectious Diseases) or Dr. Redfield's (CDC director) infectious diseases credentials, nevertheless he had a long history as a health policy expert at the Hoover Institute at Stanford University, advising presidential candidates in 2008, 2012, and 2016, as well as several members of Congress and he brought a fresh perspective to approaching the pandemic, bringing to it what I like to call the 30,000 foot view.

At the Hoover Institution, Dr. Atlas focused on public/private partnerships in health care, innovation and the impact of biotechnology, and incorporating economic factors to derive practical solutions. He was co-director there of *Socialism and Free Market Capitalism: the Human Prosperity Project.*

I knew him from his appearances on my show on Doctor Radio Reports on SiriusXM, where he also presented himself as an anti-fear monger, a non-alarmist. Unfortunately, his background as a non-virologist who was no longer seeing patients was too easily mocked by the news media, when in fact there were already plenty of virologists in the mix and not enough health policy and public health experts.

Dr. Atlas was the editor of the leading textbook in his field, *Magnetic Resonance Imaging of the Brain and Spine*, and he was chairman of neuroradiology at Stanford for many years. In this position he had trained many emerging radiologists to perform a sober analysis of an image based on pattern recognition, and he had clearly brought this ability to his career in health policy. The rationality and critical thinking needed to examine a potential brain cancer without emotion was essential to fight the fear and hysteria that has shrouded COVID. A good neuroradiologist can quickly tell you the difference on an MRI between a stroke and an abscess and a malignant versus a benign tumor.

"Throughout our friendship of more than 35 years, Dr. Atlas has always impressed with his strong expertise in analyzing public health challenges and developing concrete solutions that are based on science and data, the cornerstones of any legitimate response to COVID or other health issues," said Robert I. Grossman, MD, dean and CEO of NYU Langone Health, and a fellow, world-renowned neuroradiologist. "He has graciously stepped forward to assist with our national response to COVID, and I am confident he will contribute significantly to these efforts."

With the same kind of verisimilitude as he had shown in both medicine and health policy, Atlas was careful to distinguish between burgeoning new case numbers of COVID in Florida, Texas, and California, and the fact that the death rate wasn't climbing. He noted that children tended to have much milder cases (not always and there was the potential for serious long term complications) and that our public health priority remained to protect those most at risk. This analysis seemed prescient when, on Monday, August 17th, Florida reported 3,779 new cases on Sunday, with only 900 in Miami-Dade county, the lowest numbers since June. The numbers dropped even lower the following week.

When it came to masks, Dr. Atlas had appeared on Fox News and discussed uses and misuses. President Trump had discussed his own views on masks with me during my interview with him at the end of July. "But on the masks, my attitude is that when I was in the hospital, I felt very comfortable wearing the mask. I was seeing young people that were hurt very badly in military situations. And I felt for them, not for me, I felt for them. My wearing a mask was a good thing. I felt extremely comfortable. I don't feel comfortable in other settings when I'm all by myself on a stage and everybody's way far away. I don't think it's something that you have to do or should do, but everyone around me is tested. So I'm not the perfect person to talk about it. But I believe that you should wear it even if there's a one percent chance it helps."

Atlas agreed with this position, and suggested using masks "if you aren't able to social distance or if you are in proximity to a high risk individual." The goal according to Atlas was "stopping the deaths by protecting the high risk people. Preventing hospital overcrowding while you safely reopen society.

Dr. Deborah Birx had a more aggressive view on the role of masks, saying in Nebraska in mid August, "There is very strong evidence" that masks help control the spread of the virus, as does social distancing." In fact, recent studies had connected mask use with decreased transmission of this coronavirus in health care workers as well as in large populations.

But Atlas was disturbed by how much masks had been "highlighted and sensationalized... way out of proportion."

He was also concerned with the major role that fear was playing in public messaging throughout the pandemic. "Its stemming from a massive amount of fear bordering on hysteria. And this is a real problem because public policy is supposed to be taking into consideration not just stopping COVID-19 at all costs, but understanding the impact on people of what you do and what you say. And that's been a failure of some of the people who are speaking out on this . . . we need to live in a rational world and we need to show people that we use critical thinking . . . . the reality is there are reasons to wear a mask."

Dr. Atlas had a calm approach. He appeared to be allergic to fear mongering. He relied on data analysis and reasoning. And if he was accused of under-reacting there was certainly plenty of saber rattling around to balance him out. In fact, on the surface, he seemed to be working well with the virologists on the coronavirus task force, and was doing his best to integrate with the team.

CONCLUSION

We are afraid of the wrong things. This fear drives us to hasty observations and conclusions intended to reassure us but when not predictive over time ultimately leads to more fear. This cycle of worry is not only associated negative health outcomes like anxiety, depression, heart disease and even cancer, but in the case of COVID-19 fear it was used as a justification to imperil our entire economy and way of life.

All of it was based on a single strand of genetic material (ribonucleic acid) that utilized a spike protein on its surface to enter our cells and spread from cell to cell. Coronaviruses were not new to us—in fact at least four were in circulation as the common cold two more had led to the outbreaks of SARS in 2002 and MERS in 2012, viruses which scared us too before petering out.

But this coronavirus was far worse in terms of the symptoms it caused and as we were not fully informed by Chinese scientists, we had to learn about it as it swept through our communities. We learned in our ICUS that COVID (Coronavirus Infectious Disease) 19 caused an inflammatory response in the endothelial lining of blood vessels and throughout major organs of our body that was far worse than the direct effects of the virus itself. Lung, heart, kidney, and brain damage were common among hospitalized patients as were blood clots.

We had no control at first. We were petrified. We had few tools to fight it. No treatments. No vaccines. Our testing of the virus was delayed so we were unable to properly isolate cases and test contacts and the contagion soon became a pandemic and sped out of our control. In March we reached for anti-malarial/arthritis drug hydroxychloroquine and the antibiotic zithromax based on anecdotal evidence and studies in the lab and broad populations studies. My own father—age 96—appeared to be saved by it. But when President Trump endorsed the treatment and later admitted to taking it, it became a political hot potato and several studies showed it didn't work late in the hospital course of COVID patients. Unflawed randomized studies for early or prophylactic use were still not done (and it wasn't properly studied with zinc) but it soon became difficult to prescribe it without scrutiny (off label) amidst the politics of fear. Other studied treatments emerged for hospital use—steroids (dexamethasone), remdesivir, blood thinners, but though these treatments aided outcome, they did little to calm our fears. Convalescent plasma extracted from people who had recovered from COVID not only had a somewhat positive impact on hospitalized patients, but were also heartwarming because it meant people were giving to others, the right message to be sending to calm pandemic fears, as it is difficult to be caring and afraid at the same time. Synthetic monoclonal antibodies which targeted the SARS COV 2 virus were also emerging in the late summer which had the potential to help in serious cases.

Of course, even convalescent plasma, otherwise known as antibodies to provide passive immunity, became a political football with the election approaching in late August, 2020. For one thing, Dr. Peter Marks, director for the Center of Biologics, Evaluation, and Research at the FDA, had taken exception to some of President Trump's policies, and said he would resign if the agency "rubber stamped" an uproven COVID vaccine. Regarding plasma, Marks said "it's a strength that this was done in the real world . . . it is a weakness that we don't have a plain placebo with no plasma at all." But Marks supported the president's move (alongside FDA commissioner Dr. Stephen Hahn), "We believe that there will be enough people that will benefit from this, potentially, this being a potentially lifesaving treatment that it's worthwhile doing . . . again, we don't know for sure—that's why it's an EUA (Emergency Use Authorization).

A high level source told me that it was the leaders of the NIH who were reluctant to approve the plasma, not the FDA, because it "wasn't sexy," and hadn't been created by them, and they said hadn't been subjected to prospective double blind randomized placebo controlled clinical trials.. To me, this was politics, not science. We had been using convalescent plasma to provide passive immunity for over 100 years beginning with diptheria, polio, measles, hep B, and many other diseases, where often the treatment was given without double blinded randomized clinical trials in advance. It was a proven treatment—moderately effectiv—providing passive immunity—it was generally well tolerated with some risk of transfusion reaction and infection.

Convalescent plasma had been given to over 70,000 patients with COVID by August. The Mayo Clinic preprint (35,000 patients) showed it improved survival at 7 days and 30 days, and was especially helpful for those who received the highest amount of neutralizing antibodies.

Of course the president may have been promoting it but the reaction to him was also political and was undermining the science. Double blinded prospective randomized trials should be done but in the mean time, it was needed now for patients dying of COVID in the hospitals. It was likely somewhat effective, especially at higher doses, and many believed Dr. Marks was right that it qualified for an EUA.

An added plus was that it should increase the rate of volunteering which will increase the plasma pool. Also a good way to further test the effectiveness of immune response which is helpful for vaccine and mono-clonal antibody development.

All of this politicking around the rapidly emerging science for COVID spread more fear and uncertainty.

For prevention, we relied on a public model from 1918 even though many tried to believe it was new science. The health commissioner of St. Louis, Dr. Max Starkloff, had famously monitored the Spanish Flu outbreak in Boston and shut down his city in advance of the virus spreading to St. Louis. Schools, churches, theaters, and public gatherings were shut down, but there was a sharp uptick in deaths when the restrictions were tempo-rarily relaxed.

Employing these same mitigating strategies to decrease viral spread during COVID led to self-congratulatory messaging among public officials including Governor Cuomo when they appeared to work in New York, combined with punitive-seeming closures of schools, gyms, restaurants and churches. Protests and rallies following police murders were allowed to continue, and still the virus didn't resurge at least here in New York, proba-bly because there was little virus left in the crowds in New York to spread it by the time the protests took place beginning in early June.

We blamed others for non compliance to these old style public health methods and we blamed our leaders including President Trump for putting us in this position of millions of cases and over a hundred fifty thousand deaths by August, but we failed to blame a true culprit, the uneven unpre-pared patchwork response of entire health care system. We were simply unprepared for anything of this magnitude, a reality which we all knew deep down, a reality which generated more and more fear.

Meanwhile COVID deaths in nursing homes and around the country continued, up to 40 percent of total COVID deaths. New York was one state that had had a statute to readmit COVID positive patients to nursing homes, where the elderly were more susceptible to severe outcomes, both because of their age and other underlying medical conditions including obesity. This had led to over 6,000 COVID deaths here by late Spring.

Despite all these irregularities, Governor Cuomo was quick to blame CDC guidelines for the nursing home deaths and to cite public health measure as the reason the case count, the hospitalization rate, and the death count all dropped so dramatically in June. There was certainly much truth to this claim.

But there was another possibility that didn't receive enough attention, as the virus essentially migrated from one region to the next, ravaging a region and flooding the hospitals with patients, before moving on. This possibility had to do with cross-immunity and susceptibility.

When COVID took root, so did fear, and patients were afraid to go to the Emergency Room with non-COVID conditions and elective procedures and surgeries were cancelled. The toll on people's health and their psyche was enormous, as depression, anxiety, and suicide all mushroomed.

What we did not know DID hurt us, and we jumped to conclusions too quickly, frequently invoking the worst case scenario. COVID was an invisible mysterious killer that we couldn't see and couldn't control. Here's how the hysteria worked: *Some* asymptomatic spread quickly became in our minds *mostly* asymptomatic spread, meaning we believed the virus was everywhere on every door knob on everyone's breath. We had no proof for this but our emotional brain took over. Somehow if you wore a mask you were protected and if you didn't you were unprotected. Even if you wore a filthy mask hanging off your chin you felt some degree of protection.

If we thought we knew the problem we were also too quick to think we knew the solution—as mask wearing (rather than add to physical distancing) became the norm. Only COVID illness mattered, only COVID hospitalizations and deaths were on our radar screen. Death from suicide because of the way COVID disrupted a person's life wasn't sexy, wasn't a COVID death. Teeth that fell out or became infected because no dental care was available were somehow detachable from COVID. Heart attacks that occurred because blood pressure or cholesterol or diabetes went untreated were blurred together with COVID deaths where the heart was involved in both cases.

Schools were closed partly because of outbreaks but mostly because of COVID fears among teachers, parents, and the school administrations, legitimate when schools didn't protocol or prepare properly but somehow we failed to properly track the spread of COVID among our children outside of school. The same was true with protests—they received an automatic exemption, they were beyond our COVID radar, as though you couldn't spread the virus during an activity that was otherwise ordained.

And so we waited and hoped for an effective vaccine to stem the tide of the virus and bring us up to herd immunity. We worried about the coming Fall and flu season and weather the combination of the two killer infectious diseases would swamp our hospitals again and send us over the edge.

What had we learned? One thing we had not learned was to distinguish between emotion-driven responses and careful reasoning. We had never learned this and perhaps we can't, perhaps our brains aren't programmed this way. We certainly had learned or should have learned that we are all in this together, we are part of global health community. We can no longer think of an emerging contagion as a regional problem.

It was deeply disappointing to me that we had used COVID fears as a launching pad for divisiveness. All of us were sudden experts, hurting each other with our supposed expertise. Dogma and ridicule had presided instead of kindness and caring. It was normal to choose other strong emotions to battle our fears. But too often we had chosen negative rather than positive emotions. I am certain this can change. Courage and kindness are the best antidote to fear. Information can arm us when we have it but we need to understand that in a situation like this ferocious rapidly evolving pandemic, answers take time. Instead of respect we attacked and marginalized others. Political division was tied in to a misinformation campaign. Everyone became an expert and cherry picked who they would listen to.

Double blinded randomized controlled clinical trials were the standard, unless it was your treatment or point of view or preventative that was being touted, and then they weren't necessary. They meant that you didn't know what treatment you were getting and you could be getting a placebo. They were supposedly the gold standard of science.

Instead it was the politics of fear across the board.

Hydroxychloroquine? Rejected by the left, endorsed by the right. Prospective double blinded placebo controlled randomized trials not done.

Masking? Rejected by the right, endorsed by the left. Prospective double blinded randomized trials not done.

Effect of protests on viral spread? Endorsed by the left, rejected by the right. Prospective double blinded randomized trials not done.

Convalescent plasma? Endorsed as life saving by the right, rejected by the left for supposed lack of proof. Prospective double blinded placebo controlled randomized trials not done.

Late night comedians and political pundits drove ratings through mockery and the public listened.

This was all driven home to me the day I interviewed President Trump and he calmly and clearly presented his opinions on COVID, and also on the cognitive skills he felt were needed to be president. He appeared to me as a strong capable leader.

Person, woman, man, camera, TV were his hypotheticals of word memory. He presented them to me with his usual flare of showmanship, but they weren't a joke, he meant them seriously and I didn't interrupt him because, as Tucker Carlson later said to me on TV, I wanted to hear his answer.

But even more importantly for me, because of the way I was brought up by my two now very old parents, waiting patiently for me on their porch on Long Island, deep loving parents who taught me respect, to restrain myself and to listen to others. Beyond the 1918 public health measures we used for COVID, beyond emerging treatments and a spectacularly produced vaccine, our best tool against our fears was two words. Respect and kindness. Kindness and respect.

Former Vice President Biden sounded like a healer too when he accepted the Democratic nomination for president on August 20th. He talked about restoring the "soul of America" and delivering us from darkness. He spoke about protecting us and getting a handle on the coronavirus pandemic in part with increased testing and daily briefings. Compassion and hope were two key words in his speech, which though it was read from a teleprompter, was nevertheless strong and projecting leadership, a treatment for fear.

But the problem for me and many others was that he talked much too quickly about national mandates and the potential for more lockdowns, which may have helped somewhat in the early going but were also sucking the soul out of America, its businesses and its people. Plus, it wasn't clear that public health measures, even less drastic ones like contact tracing, distancing and masking were the entire answer here. The virus seemed to be ravaging certain areas, especially highly congested socio-economically disadvantaged areas, before moving on. It wasn't herd immunity exactly, but there definitely seemed to be more T cell and humoral (antibody) immunity in these regions than we were able to document, including perhaps partial immunity from other coronaviruses. There was also the distinct possibility that the virus was mutating (or could mutate) into a less virulent form, which could help explain why the death and hospitalization rates were down (plus a higher percentage of younger people being affected, who tended to have milder cases).

Dr. Anthony Fauci was clearly one of the top virologists and vaccinologists in the world and had been so for a long time. But his expertise and messaging on lockdowns and severe restrictions left something to be desired. When he spoke to me about it on Doctor Radio he was more nuanced about the great public health costs as well as the limitations.

At the time of this writing, there were 24 million documented COVID-19 cases in the world, with 822,000 deaths. In the U.S. there were 5.85 million cases, with 180,000 deaths from COVID, and the real numbers of cases (unreported) were likely much higher. Surgeon General Vice Admiral Dr. Adams tweeted out on August 27th, 2020 that cases were trending down by 14 percent, test positivity down one percent, hospitalizations down 11 percent, and deaths down over 8 percent. But that day there was still over 40,000 new cases, and over a thousand deaths in the country from COVID. We still had a long long way to go. The virus had attacked New York first, our nerve and media center, sounding every alarm possible before moving on. But in late August we were still captivated by it, we were learning more every day about long term complications, and we still lived in a world of fear.

On Doctor Radio on SiriusXM on August 25th, 2020, I as the medical director, on my regular show, Doctor Radio Reports; Coronavirus, What You Need to Know Right Now, interviewed Dr. Jeffrey Lieberman, Chairman of the Department of Psychiatry at Columbia Presbyterian Medical Center told me that a "tsunami of psychiatric sequelae is looming which will roil the American population. A psychological disruption to our whole society," he said. I knew he was right, and I stayed up at night trying to figure out what we could do about it. During the day I donned my N95 mask and gown, shield and gloves, and returned to the office, sometimes seeing nervous patients who had been exposed to COVID but continuing to test negative myself. New York seemed soulless, fearful, masked survivors lining the streets, but at least the virus was mostly gone.

Back at the end of July I had given the two words "respect and kindness "out to Tucker Carlson's audience of millions as my prescription two days after my interview with President Trump. He had shown me respect and kindness at the White House and whatever people thought of him or of me for that matter, I wanted everyone to know those two words and to try them out on each other.

Taking the high road provided a vaccine not for the virus itself but for the fear it spawned.

RESOURCES

PART 1

Siegel, M. (2006). *False Alarm: The Truth about the Epidemic of Fear.* John Wiley & Sons.

Siegel, M. (2006). *Bird flu: Everything you need to know about the next pandemic.* Hoboken, N.J: Wiley

www.ncbi.nlm.nih.gov/pmc/articles/PMC4119830

hms.harvard.edu/news/covid-blood-type

www.sciencemag.org/news/2020/07/school-openings

medicalxpress.com/news/2020-07-commentary-pediatrics-children-dont-transmit.html

www.healthdata.org/covid/updates

jamanetwork.com/journals/jamacardiology/fullarticle/2768916

jamanetwork.com/journals/jamacardiology/fullarticle/2768915

www.sciencemag.org/news/2020/07/brain-fog-heart-damage-covid-19-s-lingering-problems-alarm-scientists

wwwnc.cdc.gov/eid/article/12/1/05-0965_article

www.cdc.gov/measles/about/history.html

www.nejm.org/doi/full/10.1056/NEJMoa2022483

www.nejm.org/doi/full/10.1056/NEJMoa2024671

www.research.ox.ac.uk/Article/2020-07-19-the-oxford-covid-19-vaccine

blogs.sciencemag.org/pipeline/archives/2020/08/06/vaccine-data-from

www.globaltimes.cn/content/1197911.shtml

www.ncbi.nlm.nih.gov/pmc/articles/PMC7284272

www.ncbi.nlm.nih.gov/pmc/articles/PMC7177048

www.ncbi.nlm.nih.gov/books/NBK92479

www.cdc.gov/flu/avianflu/h5n1-people.htm

www.fiercebiotech.com/biotechall-three-novartis-a-h1n1-2009-influenza
-vaccines-prequalified-by-world-health-organization

www.cidrap.umn.edu/news-perspective/2009/09/fda-approves-four
-companies-h1n1-vaccines

thehill.com/policy/healthcare/513106-new-ebola-outbreak-in-congo
-raises-alarm

thehill.com/opinion/healthcare/473805-deadly-measles-and-ebola
-outbreaks-show-why-vaccinations-are-so-essential

www.nytimes.com/2014/07/28/world/africa/ebola-epidemic-west-africa
-guinea.html

www.thelancet.com/journals/lancet/article/PIIS0140-6736(14)61428-8/
fulltext

www.governing.com/news/headlines/texas-health-officials-watching-up
-to-100-people-in-connection-with-ebola-case.html

www.kff.org/news-summary/up-to-10000-ebola-orphans-face-stigma
-in-west-africa/

www.doctorswithoutborders.org/what-we-do/news-stories/research/
report-ebola-2014-2015-facts-and-figures

www.latimes.com/business/la-fi-frontier-airline-ebola-patient-20141015
-story.html

www.dallasnews.com/news/2016/02/defect-causing-zika-virus-found
-in-dallas-county.html/

slate.com/technology/2005/09/don-t-worry-be-healthy.html

www.cbsnews.com/news/nih-doctor-explains-u-s-efforts-to-combat
-zika-virus

www.newsweek.com/expect-us-zika-outbreak-summer-says-top-health
-official-448761

www.cdc.gov/zika/pdfs/control_mosquitoes_chikv_denv_zika.pdf

www.sciencedaily.com/releases/2017/03/170324104927.htm

www.cdc.gov/mmwr/volumes/65/wr/mm6530e1.htm

www.cdc.gov/dengue/about

www.statnews.com/2019/05/01/fda-dengue-vaccine-restrictions

www.cdc.gov/mmwr/volumes/65/wr/mm6524e2.htm

www.ncbi.nlm.nih.gov/pmc/articles/PMC6062015

www.statnews.com/2016/09/28/senate-approves-zika-funding

slate.com/technology/2016/04/a-zika-outbreak-in-the-u-s-is-not-anything
-to-panic-about.html

www.newscientist.com/article/2088612-cancel-the-olympic-games-in
 -brazil-because-of-zika-no-way
slate.com/technology/2016/08/zika-is-spreading-in-florida-but-we-know
 -how-to-stop-it.html
www.foxnews.com/opinion/zika-virus-fear-facts-and-the-future
www.nih.gov/news-events/news-releases/nih-developed-zika-vaccine
 -improves-fetal-outcomes-animal-model
www.nature.com/articles/s41541-020-0167-8?utm_source=feedbur
 ner&utm_medium=feed&utm_campaign=Feed%3A+npjvaccines%-
 2Frss%2Fcurrent+%28npj+Vaccines%29

PART 2

www.nbcnews.com/health/health-news/live-blog/2020-03-07-coronavirus
 -news-n1152081
www.southampton.ac.uk/news/2020/03/covid-19-china.page
www.who.int/dg/speeches/detail/who-director-general-s-remarks-at-the
 -media-briefing-on-2019-ncov-on-10-february-2020
www.whitehouse.gov/presidential-actions/proclamation-suspension
 -entry-immigrants-nonimmigrants-persons-pose-risk-transmit-
 ting-2019-novel-coronavirus
www.fmprc.gov.cn/mfa_eng/zxxx_662805/t1737014.shtml
www.wsj.com/articles/world-health-coronavirus-disinformation
 -11586122093
www.who.int/dg/speeches/detail/who-director-general-s-statement-on
 -the-advice-of-the-ihr-emergency-committee-on-novel-coronavirus
www.theweek.in/news/world/2020/05/13/covid-19-after-german
 -intelligence-now-cia-believes-china-tried-to-coerce-who.html
www.foxnews.com/world/world-health-organization-january-tweet
 -china-human-transmission-coronavirus
.www.fda.gov/news-events/press-announcements/coronavirus-covid-19
 -update-daily-roundup-march-30-2020
www.nature.com/articles/s41421-020-0156-0
jamanetwork.com/journals/jama/fullarticle/2766117
www.abc.net.au/news/2020-06-05/hydroxychloroquine-study-the
 -lancet-peer-review-coronavirus/12324118
www.acpjournals.org/doi/10.7326/M20-4207

www.nejm.org/doi/full/10.1056/NEJMoa2019014

www.nejm.org/doi/full/10.1056/NEJMoa2016638

www.nejm.org/doi/full/10.1056/NEJMe2020388

coronavirus.health.ny.gov/covid-19-travel-advisory

www.billboard.com/articles/news/awards/9439819/new-york-mandatory
-quarantine-rules-vmas-talent

www.stltoday.com/news/resolute-doctor-protected-st-louis-max-starkloff
-s-insistence-on/article_d7694b21-e8d5-539f-b87e-acfd5fa3ec90.html

www.nebraskamed.com/COVID/spreading-facts-to-fight-the-coronavirus

www.bbc.com/news/world-asia-53274085

www.nytimes.com/2020/08/04/us/virus-testing-delays.html

www.wsj.com/articles/a-state-by-state-guide-to-coronavirus-lockdowns
-11584749351 blogs.imf.org/2020/04/14/the-great-lockdown-worst
-economic-downturn-since-the-great-depression/

journals.plos.org/plosmedicine/article?id=10.1371/journal.pmed
.1003166

www.smithsonianmag.com/history/philadelphia-threw-wwi-parade-gave
-thousands-onlookers-flu-180970372

www.psychiatrictimes.com/view/spanish-flu-pandemic-and-mental-health
-historical-perspective

www.psychiatry.org/newsroom/news-releases/apa-reaffirms-support-for
-goldwater-rule

yaledailynews.com/blog/2020/05/13/profile-dr-bandy-lee-and-the
-psychiatric-case-against-donald-trump/

www.healthaffairs.org/doi/10.1377/hlthaff.2020.00818?utm_medium
=press&utm_source=mediaadvisory&utm_campaign=covidfasttrack
&utm_content=lyu

www.cdc.gov/media/releases/2020/p0714-americans-to-wear-masks.html

www.cnbc.com/2020/08/13/trump-calls-bidens-coronavirus-plan
-unscientific-rejects-call-for-national-mask-mandate.html

www.usatoday.com/story/opinion/2020/06/30/coronavirus-wear
-masks-socially-distance-new-lockdowns-column/3274637001/

www.insider.com/wear-face-masks-during-sex-prevent-coronavirus-spread
-harvard-study-2020-6

thehill.com/homenews/state-watch/511483-wisconsin-state-agency
-requires-employees-to-wear-masks-while

www.nature.com/articles/s41591-020-0843-2

www.acpjournals.org/doi/10.7326/M20-1342

www.sciencealert.com/40-of-people-with-covid-19-don-t-have-symptoms
-latest-cdc-estimate-says

file:///Users/marcsiegel/Downloads/WHO-2019-nCov-IPC_Masks-2020
.4-eng.pdf

www.hhs.gov/about/news/2020/07/22/us-government-engages-pfizer
-produce-millions-doses-covid-19-vaccine.html

www.nejm.org/doi/full/10.1056/nejmoa2022483

www.pfizer.com/news/press-release/press-release-detail/pfizer-and
-biontech-choose-lead-mrna-vaccine-candidate-0

www.nejm.org/doi/full/10.1056/NEJMoa2024671

www.thelancet.com/journals/lancet/article/PIIS0140-6736(20)31604-4/
fulltext

www.worldpharmanews.com/research/5339-single-shot-covid-19-vaccine
-protects-non-human-primates

www.statnews.com/2020/07/07/novavax-maker-of-a-covid-19-vaccine-is
-backed-by-operation-warp-speed/

www.wsj.com/articles/novavax-covid-19-vaccine-produces-positive-results
-in-first-stage-study-11596571200

www.sciencemag.org/news/2020/08/russia-s-approval-covid-19-vaccine
-less-meets-press-release

www.theguardian.com/world/2020/aug/20/global-report-who-in-talks
-with-russia-over-covid-19-vaccine

www.nature.com/articles/d41586-020-02244-1

www.ncbi.nlm.nih.gov/pmc/articles/PMC7177048

www.ncbi.nlm.nih.gov/pmc/articles/PMC7284272

www.nbcnews.com/politics/2020-election/poll-less-half-americans-say
-they-ll-get-coronavirus-vaccine-n1236971

www.sciencemag.org/news/2020/06/just-50-americans-plan-get-covid-19
-vaccine-here-s-how-win-over-rest

ttps://news.gallup.com/poll/317018/one-three-americans-not-covid
-vaccine.aspx

www.baltimoresun.com/coronavirus/ct-nw-nyt-covid-19-vaccine-race
-20200709-37nkwjzk6reypp6d3alkazy34u-story.html

www.nejm.org/doi/full/10.1056/NEJMsa2011686

www.nimh.nih.gov/news/science-news/2020/nimh-directors-statement
-on-racism.shtml

news.osu.edu/covid-19-update-university-shares-return-to-campus
-updates-testing-program-expansion/

www.thelantern.com/2020/08/letter-to-the-editor-ohio-state-should
-reevaluate-opening-campus-this-fall/www.ksro.com/2020/08/16/
coronavirus-updates-unc-chapel-hill-has-4th-cluster-of-cases-in-3-
days/

www.wflx.com/2020/08/17/florida-case-increase-lowest-months-deaths
-rise-by

www.medscape.com/viewarticle/936180

www.nytimes.com/interactive/2020/us/coronavirus-us-cases.html

www.azcentral.com/story/news/local/arizona-health/2020/08/18/maricopa
-county-many-phoenix-area-cities-still-require-mask-now/
3360523001/

www.azcentral.com/story/opinion/op-ed/laurieroberts/2020/08/19/gov
-doug-ducey-has-chance-save-face-and-mandate-masks/3393827001/

azgovernor.gov/governor/news/2020/07/governor-ducey-issues-executive
-order-further-protect-public-health

www.marketwatch.com/story/sweden-has-developed-herd-immunity-after
-refusing-to-lock-down-experts-claim-its-coronavirus-infection-rate
-is-falling-2020-08-24

coronavirus.jhu.edu/data/new-cases

labornotes.org/2020/07/full-steam-ahead-reopening-schools-no-way-say
-teachers

www.silive.com/coronavirus/2020/08/nyc-teachers-push-for-schools-to
-stay-closed-come-fall.html

www.nytimes.com/interactive/2020/07/31/us/coronavirus-school
-reopening-risk.html

www.reuters.com/article/us-coronavirus-health-education-nebraska/
nebraska-school-district-cancels-classes-as-staff-catch-coronavirus
-idUSKCN25C067

wwwnc.cdc.gov/eid/article/26/10/20-1315_article

www.sciencedaily.com/releases/2020/08/200804100225.htm

www.sciencemag.org/news/2020/07/school-openings-across-globe
-suggest-ways-keep-coronavirus-bay-despite-outbreaks

www.cdc.gov/mmwr/volumes/69/wr/mm6932e3.htm

www.cidrap.umn.edu/news-perspective/2020/08/cdcs-redfield-addresses
-school-reopening-citing-promising-study

www.cdc.gov/mmwr/volumes/69/wr/mm6934e2.htm

www.cdc.gov/mmwr/volumes/69/wr/mm6932a1.htm

today.duke.edu/2020/08/keeping-close-watch-covid-19-surveillance-tests

news.cornell.edu/stories/2020/08/surveillance-testing-set-begin-sept-2

cornellsun.com/2020/08/09/in-a-rocky-start-to-august-students-scramble
    -to-make-quarantine-plans/

www.southbendtribune.com/news/local/notre-dame-sees-spike-in-covid
    -19-cases/article_df400178-de64-11ea-9eec-8f4e8e14e00d.html

www.cbsnews.com/news/notre-dame-covid-cases-off-campus-party
    -classes-suspended/

www.nytimes.com/2020/08/18/us/notre-dame-coronavirus.html

www.dailytarheel.com/article/2020/08/breaking-dashboard-update-0817

news.osu.edu/covid-19-update-university-shares-return-to-campus
    -updates-testing-program-expansion/

www.thelantern.com/2020/08/letter-to-the-editor-ohio-state-should
    -reevaluate-opening-campus-this-fall/

www.ksro.com/2020/08/16/coronavirus-updates-unc-chapel-hill-has
    -4th-cluster-of-cases-in-3-days/

www.southbendtribune.com/news/local/notre-dame-sees-spike-in-covid
    -19-cases/article_df400178-de64-11ea-9eec-8f4e8e14e00d.html

www.cdc.gov/coronavirus/2019-ncov/community/colleges-universities/
    considerations.html

www.cdc.gov/coronavirus/2019-ncov/community/colleges-universities/
    index.html

www.marketwatch.com/story/as-pandemic-rages-prominent-colleges
    -announce-online-semesters-11594130062

www.insidehighered.com/news/2020/08/12/hundreds-colleges-walk
    -back-fall-reopening-plans-and-opt-online-only-instruction

www.columbiaspectator.com/spectrum/2020/08/14/this-just-in
    -columbia-is-entirely-online-for-undergraduates-mostly-online
    -for-graduate-students/

globalnews.ca/news/7131010/coronavirus-canada-students-gap-year

www.theverge.com/2020/8/17/21371999/college-startups-pandemic-coro-
    navirus-covid19-internships-fall

www.npr.org/2020/07/21/893221346/when-can-kids-go-back-to-school
    -leaders-say-as-soon-as-it-s-safe

www.cdc.gov/media/releases/2020/t0205-coronavirus-update.html

www.siriusxm.com/clips/clip/e7adfb79-ca09-4825-b8ca-1aa0c124dea0/
    d9f802c7-1bdc-443f-8034-d119f322468b

www.hhs.gov/about/news/2020/03/13/secretary-azar-designates
    -admiral-giroir-coordinate-covid-19-diagnostic-testing-efforts.html

www.fda.gov/news-events/press-announcements/coronavirus-covid-19
    -update-daily-roundup-august-3-2020

www.bbc.com/news/world-latin-america-52711458

www.nytimes.com/interactive/2020/world/asia/india-coronavirus
    -cases.html

ourworldindata.org/coronavirus-testing

www.nature.com/articles/s41581-020-0327-0

www.cell.com/action/showPdf?pii=S2666-3791%2820%2930102-6

newsroom.uw.edu/news/antibodies-block-sars-cov-2-infection
    -fishing-crew

bearingdrift.com/2019/09/11/the-9-11-bullhorn-speech-by-president
    -george-w-bush-2

myfox8.com/news/washington-dc-bureau/white-house-releases-new
    -report-president-used-defense-production-act-nearly-80-times-to
    -combat-pandemic/

thehill.com/homenews/state-watch/489214-cuomo-says-ny-needs-30000
    -ventilators-pleads-with-feds-for-help

nypost.com/2020/05/01/javits-center-hospital-to-close-after-treating
    -1000-patients/

www.governor.ny.gov/news/governor-cuomo-announces-covid-19
    -infection-rate-below-1-percent-tenth-straight-day

www.syracuse.com/coronavirus/2020/08/cuomo-official-grilled-on
    -coronavirus-nursing-home-deaths-secrecy.html

www.medscape.com/viewarticle/935666

www.hrsa.gov/CovidUninsuredClaim

www.cdc.gov/coronavirus/2019-ncov/prevent-getting-sick/how-covid
    -spreads.html

update.covid19.ca.gov

www.news4jax.com/news/florida/2020/08/21/floridas-positive-covid-19
    -test-rate-trends-down-over-last-week/

www.nytimes.com/2020/08/07/opinion/coronavirus-lockdown
    -unemployment-death.html

www.politico.com/news/2020/08/17/biden-contemplated-suicide
    -after-1972-deaths-wife-daughter-397487

www.statnews.com/2020/08/20/ramped-up-testing-and-daily-briefings
    -inside-bidens-plan-to-take-over-the-governments-tumultuous-covid
    -19-response/
www.marketwatch.com/story/trumps-new-hire-to-coronavirus-task-force
    -lacks-infectious-disease-expertise-opposes-shutdowns-2020-08-16
www.hoover.org/profiles/scott-w-atlas
www.chicagotribune.com/coronavirus/ct-nw-trump-scott-atlas
    -coronavirus-20200816-kp5mmxr2ibfqppquppxtb3kko4-story.html
profiles.stanford.edu/scott-atlas
video.foxnews.com/v/6180318434001?playlist_d=5198073478001#sp
    =show-clips
www.medscape.com/viewarticle/935666
journalstar.com/lifestyles/health-med-fit/during-nebraska-visit-dr
    -birx-says-masks-should-not-be-a-partisan-issue/article
    _290c7eec-b633-5a1e-8a57-56426dbfc20a.html

CONCLUSION

www.cdc.gov/coronavirus/general-information.html
www.who.int/news-room/fact-sheets/detail/middle-east-respiratory
    -syndrome-coronavirus-(mers-cov)
www.ncbi.nlm.nih.gov/pmc/articles/PMC7229726
www.thelancet.com/journals/lanhae/article/PIIS2352-3026(20)30216-7/
    fulltext
www.pharmaceutical-technology.com/comment/dexamethasone
    -remdesivir-combination-covid/
www.fda.gov/emergency-preparedness-and-response/coronavirus
    -disease-2019-covid-19/donate-covid-19-plasma
www.nih.gov/news-events/news-releases/clinical-trials-monoclonal
    -antibodies-prevent-covid-19-now-enrolling
www.reuters.com/article/us-health-coronavirus-vaccines-fda-exclu/
    exclusive-top-fda-official-says-would-resign-if-agency-rubber-stamps
    -an-unproven-covid-19-vaccine-idUSKBN25H03H
abcnews.go.com/Health/fda-issue-emergency-authorization-convalescent
    -plasma-treatment-hospitalized/story?id=72556828
www.medrxiv.org/content/10.1101/2020.08.12.20169359v1
www.nationalgeographic.com/history/2020/03/how-cities-flattened
    -curve-1918-spanish-flu-pandemic-coronavirus/

www.usatoday.com/story/opinion/voices/2020/07/22/andrew-cuomo
-nursing-homes-coronavirus-janice-dean-new-york-column/
5472713002

www.nature.com/articles/s41577-020-0389-z

www.ncbi.nlm.nih.gov/pmc/articles/PMC7276840

www.foxnews.com/politics/joe-biden-accepts-democratic-presidential
-nomination-closes-out-four-day-virtual-convention.

www.nytimes.com/interactive/2020/us/coronavirus-us-cases.html

covid.cdc.gov/covid-data-tracker/?CDC_AA_refVal=https%3A%2F
%2F

cdc.gov%2Fcoronavirus%2F2019-ncov%2Fcases-updates%2Fcounty-map
.html#county-map